ADRIAN GRIST

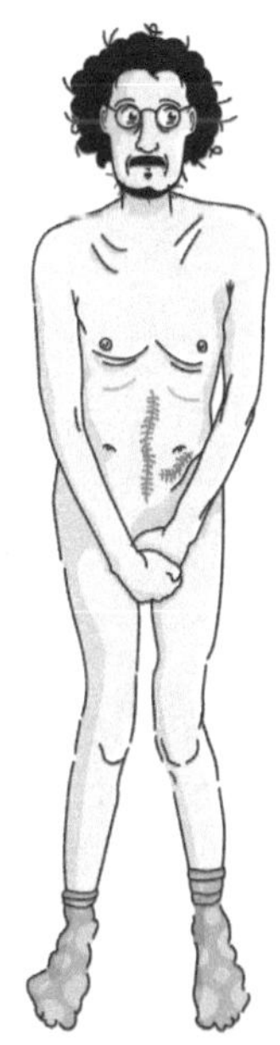

TRANSPLANTED & EXPOSED

ISBN 978-91-527-3601-2
Published by Adrian Grist

This book contains the recollections and memories of the author as they were perceived at the time.
The author is aware that he was on a bucketload of painkillers and a cocktail of drugs during some of the events recalled, and that he also has impaired vision. Bear that in mind if you were present and perceived things differently. In the main, real names are used other than when there is a real risk of litigation or job loss.

All artwork by Will Gray
Author photo by Robin Moore

To the Swedish Wife, Mum
and the chap who died
at the age of 19
without whom this book would never
have been written

CONTENTS

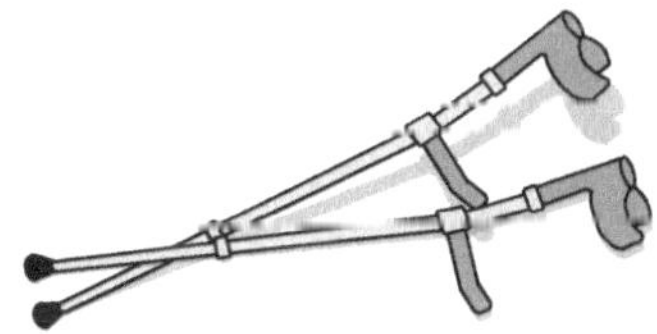

Foreword

This book wasn't even my idea. If I were ever to have a forte, then it'd probably be 'missing the blindingly obvious'. There are two reasons for this: firstly, as a white man born in the United Kingdom and raised within the blurry boundaries of the middle-classes, it is almost nigh-on impossible to escape a cosseted and privileged upbringing. Such formative years render you blinkered from the extremes of society, or indeed anything which is going on outside your cosy, cushioned bubble. My upbringing was far from privileged, but as a slightly more world-weary grownup, I can certainly reflect on quite how lucky I was. I wasn't born with a silver spoon in my mouth, not in the slightest, but there was some silver cutlery in the sideboard which was dusted off for special occasions.

Secondly, the word 'blindingly' contains the word 'blind'. While I was born with fully functioning eyes and 20/20 vision, late in my teens a diagnosis led me onto a path which ultimately required me to undergo six surgeries to save my eyesight. I have since been left with seriously depleted peripheral vision and the inability to distinguish colours or even my own wife from over seven metres away.

Spotting both 'new perspectives' and 'uncovered manholes' therefore requires some assistance. It was my colleague, Ellen, who, back in March 2020, reflected on my personal circumstances and suggested I document my experiences as the corona pandemic went from its embryonic stages to being a healthy, bouncing bundle of wanton death and destruction.

The 'personal circumstances' to which she was referring

form the narrative of this book. My life has been ravaged by disease and various disorders, which ultimately rendered me as odds-on favourite to snuff it at the spiky hands of any virus, never mind the now infamous SARS-CoV-2.

In addition to this, I have dual citizenship with two countries which were at total odds in regard to how to tackle a pandemic. The government of the country I now live in told me to do one thing, and the government of the country in which I was born told me to do the polar opposite.

I knew from the start that self-publishing might very well be the only way to get my story heard, and I knew that might mean that only my wife and my mum would end up buying it – and they are both already overfamiliar with these tales of woe and wooziness in all their gory and grizzly detail. If you find yourself holding this book and you are neither my wife nor my mum, then I cannot tell you how grateful I am to you.

This book might get a bit piss-y, poo-y, icky, sicky, bile-y and bloody, but my intention isn't really to offend or make you feel uncomfortable. And this book is not about the pandemic per se, but rather it is meant as a window on, and exploration of, a life being lived with hidden disabilities.

Also, I am painfully aware that in the latter stages of the book, my genitals might dominate proceedings. I know the world does not need another man talking about his knob in a public forum, but it really is a pivotal point of the narrative, so there it stays.

Finally, I am just one speck on the spectrum of disability, but I am a speck who is afforded both the luxury of time and inclination to share my story. I know it is revolting, but I also hope you'll find it revealing, refreshingly honest and hopefully funny.

Chapter 1
Reborn in a pandemic

Friday, May 15th, 2009.

I think I've shit myself. *Have I shit myself?* It wouldn't have been the first time – and it has turned out not to be the last. But this time, I was in a room seemingly full of people, and I knew I had to tell someone.

The reality was that I had never knowingly entered that room, and I have no recollection of ever leaving it. It was a recovery room where I was flitting in and out consciousness after a ten-hour-plus stint under the collective scalpels of a team of surgeons.

(And it wasn't an entirely unfounded thought, I'd been making a bit of a habit of soiling sheets in the months running up to this moment.)

I had just undergone a double organ transplant, during which – and I say this as someone who never even opted to take biology as a high school subject – I had, as I was later informed, lost more blood than the average adult male has circulating in his body. Having said that, I had so many blood transfusions in the previous year, I am not quite sure how much of that blood was mine to lose in the first place.

If I'd really thought about it, there was no way I could have actually shit myself, as I'd had a bowel-emptying enema hours before going under the knife. An hour before that, I had thrown up the moment I had put the phone down after hearing the words, 'we think we have matching organs for you'. If that wasn't enough, I gagged up any remnants of bile in a lay-by in the small village of Great Chesterford en route to the hospital in Cambridge. There was no doubt about it, I was empty – not a scrap or drop left to poo or puke. I couldn't have pissed myself either, for that matter. I hadn't pissed for a few years by this point. I had my first piss for a long time a few days after this operation. Weird how one can forget how annoying having to go for a piss actually can be.

Either way, that was the first thought of my salvaged life: 'I think I have shit myself.' I could make out the fast-moving green scrubs of the people pouring over me as I uttered the thought out loud. I felt something being shoved underneath me; maybe they suspected I was telling the truth, although no one could've known better than a team of surgeons who had just spent an entire shift rifling through my guts just how empty I actually was.

*****

The next few days were spent in a high dependency ward. I was told if the operation had gone badly, I'd have been in intensive care, although I could not figure how the care could be any more intensive than what I was receiving.

A nurse sat at the end of my bed. I cannot recall her face, only faint scraps of her voice. She would perform the regular vital statistics tests I had become horribly familiar with over the last decade, although the blood pressure cuff would give me a tough-love squeeze with alarming regularity. On top of all that, she had a new trick up her sleeve – one which felt like it might have been a request for a more sexually deviant patient whose notes had somehow got muddled up with mine. At least a couple of times a day, she'd come to my bed with an ice cube and run it from nipple height down my torso, not lifting it from the skin as she passed my groin and down to my inner thigh. I couldn't feel a thing, so from an erotic perspective, an epic fail. I later established that me 'not feeling a thing' was what she was hoping for, as a 'thing' is not what you want to be feeling when you have been effectively sawn in two then stitched and stapled back together again. She was simply testing that the epidural pain block was working its numbing magic.

There was a line into the main artery in my neck, from which the blood-testing chap could open a tap and drain me with the apparent ease of an experienced barperson pouring a pint of Guinness. I had three cannulas in each arm, two tubes which felt as cumbersome as garden hoses protruding from either side of my abdomen, and a feeding line which mystifyingly seemed to go into my lungs. I also had a catheter shoved up my willy which, through no one's fault, caused such trauma I would within the year find myself back under the knife having a circumcision. (Reflecting on this, I have an uncle who has nagged me about paying greater homage to my supposed Jewish roots, but for the record, I consider this as far as that homage will ever go). I also had an oxygen mask, but do you really count something which does not penetrate through your skin when totting up the number of anatomical intruders? Everything was attached to either a pulsating/bleeping machine or a slowly emptying/slowly filling bag of piss, bile or highly calorific 'food'.

And I felt abso-bloody-lutely amazing.

I could not remember feeling this good. The statistic they use to gauge kidney function was racing towards 'healthy'. I could feel the energy pump into my body minute by minute, hour by hour. My sugar levels, which had only a day before erratically rocketed then crashed, were steadying themselves at a comfortable cruising healthy altitude.

But to truly contextualise the dizzying heights of feeling 'abso-bloody-lutely amazing', one must first consider the dismal depths from which I rose.

When the downward spiral of ill health takes up almost a decade of a life, one has myriad examples of quite how bad it all can get. One of the early low points was when a chronic bone disorder resulted in me having to wear a cast on one foot and a medical plastic boot on the other. For over a year. That bone condition, and subsequent treatment, has left me – and these words have genuinely appeared on my medical files – 'acutely deformed'.

The impact of my organ failure resulted in dwindling vision, which announced itself with a sudden leak of blood at the back of my retina. It blinded me in one eye while I was attending a dinner party. It felt too rude to spoil the mood, so I kept it quiet; we had already commenced with dessert, so no need to ruin things now. I used one eye to drive home and made a hospital appointment for 'as soon as you possibly can, please. Just help me ... *please*'.

In the end, both eyes needed months of painful laser treatment and – as it now stands – six operations to stabilise my sight. During the early, blurry months I would wake up not knowing what I would be able to see as I opened my eyes. The blood at the back of my retinas acted almost like a child's kaleidoscope; day by day, what I could see changed. I did as much as I possibly could on a good day. On a bad day, I had about five per cent vision through which I could just about watch daytime telly.

However, the behemoth of all lows was being on dialysis for more than a year. I was painfully aware, both figuratively and literally, of the trajectory my ill health was likely to plummet. The hard-fought battle to save my kidney function, which had raged for around two years, was clearly being lost (unless you were on the side of 'kidney failure').

The increasingly large, black swirls of blood in my eyes meant that more and more of my days were spent watching telly through a pinprick of light. While I was not a wheelchair user all of the time, I was certainly more manoeuvrable if I could be rolled. So most trips out of the house (hospital or supermarket) were on four wheels.

There were moments when I considered the tipping point of my physical ability – would there be a time when I might become so helpless that I could not execute an exit strategy with a lethal injection of the cocktail of drugs I had chilling in my fridge? After each debilitating blow my body received, I'd find myself reconfiguring that plan, and I felt confident that I could navigate my broken and blind body from my upstairs bedroom to the kitchen where I could crank up a permanent nightcap.

While I cannot believe now that this was ever a consideration, it *is* in my memory, so I guess it must have been. Although, the fact that I was blind, crippled, and facing dialysis for an indeterminate period and yet maintaining relatively good cheer would suggest a one-way hobble downstairs was not likely to happen.

*****

So, peritoneal dialysis it was for me. If there was ever a marketing campaign for the joys of peritoneal dialysis, it would be targeted at the 'dynamic, professional, go-getter'. It would almost certainly feature a busy, working mother being portrayed giving a presentation in a board room, smashing an ace against a male tennis opponent, and then enjoying an early evening mocktail with her besties.

(Haemodialysis is what most people think of when they think of dialysis machines. That's the one where you have to go into hospital every other day and sit next to a giant machine while it gives your blood a thorough rinsing. It's definitely the 'less sexy' of the two options, as if there is anything remotely sexy about peritoneal dialysis whatsoever – it was certainly not a fetish my then girlfriend was into, I know that at least.)

It basically meant, at least in my case, that I could dialyse overnight from the comfort of my own home. I was becoming au fait and okay about my increasing housebound status and didn't relish the alternative of having to leave those comforts every second day for haemodialysis, where I'd be plumbed into a something, which, to my mind, resembled a contraption from a sci-fi B-movie set. This way, I'd never need to be more than a crawl away from my own toilet, kettle, and fridge-stored suicide ingredients – perfect!

(I did a lot of crawling when I had one foot in a cast and another in a medical boot. I could take the latter off easily, but it was a tad tricky to put back on. Sometimes it just felt easier to crawl than to reassemble myself, and it did not take me long to learn to adeptly ascend stairs on my knees and descend them on my bum).

Peritoneal dialysis uses the inside lining of your abdomen as a filter. It's all rather science-y, and at that point in my life, I didn't even have the concentration power to formulate a shopping list, let alone bother with researching the machinations of dialysis.

Before treatment started, an incision was made just south of my belly button, and a tube was fed into the space in my gut where I had previously thought I had stored 'fart'. During the day, when the tube was not in use, it would be taped to my tummy – a period of my life when I reverted to a baggy jumper grunge teen look to disguise the protrusion.

The insertion of the tube is considered a relatively straightforward procedure, which can be done in twenty minutes or so under sedation and local anaesthetic. It was, however, only after two botched attempts – including one where I woke up mid-procedure – that we struck third time 'lucky'. It was early in 2008 that I was set on a path which could only end in two ways – dialysis until death or someone else dying and me snaffling their organs for a transplant. Either way, someone's mum was going to be very upset indeed. At this point, both my kidneys and my pancreas were banjaxed beyond repair.

My medical supplies were so weighty and cumbersome that they arrived in an articulated lorry with a pneumatic loading ramp. It took a burly man around fifteen round trips to bring in all the boxes and lug them upstairs. They were stored in a bedroom which had only been deemed 'spare' after a housemate who rented the room from me was asked to leave just to afford me the space this new lifestyle required. At one point, I genuinely feared the weight of the supplies would cause structural damage to the house. Bags of fluids in boxes, which lined all four walls, were piled up to the ceiling; beyond that were litres and litres of cleaning supplies and various tubes to connect this to that, and that to me.

A nurse came to my home and spent five days training me on how to set up the machine. It works by pumping in the dialysing fluids through the pipe into my peritoneal cavity. There the fluid sat and did its science-y stuff, before being extracted via the same tube and then directed into a 'piss bag' (not a term the nurse used) which lay next to my bed. It worked in cycles and took about ten litres to do the job in total. In the morning, I would drag the bag of piss downstairs and empty it in the bath.

The nurse lectured me on the importance of good hand hygiene long before it was 'trendy'. I was taught and then tested on how to scrub up properly, which, if done correctly, would take three minutes. To make the whole process more 'fun', she gave me a novelty egg timer shaped like a chicken.

A chicken. Nothing quite distracts you from your depressing lived reality quite like a plastic chicken. Hygiene was of the utmost importance, so I never had the heart to tell her that my cat would curl up and doze on the warm dialysis machine. Nor that he got infinitely more use out of the chicken than I ever did.

The lows will follow, but the everydays and standouts included ...

not being able to drink more than one and a half litres of fluid a day, washing with alcohol wipes instead of showering, never being able to spend a night away from home, taking more than 40 pills a day, having to inject myself five times a day, my cat waking me up by playing with the tube which vibrated as it pumped fluid in me, the time the piss bag broke and I woke up with seven litres of urine-reeking discharge on the carpet which actually created a wet patch on the ceiling of the room below, a heavily restricted diet which ruled out most fresh fruit and vegetables, missing weddings, bailing on friends' birthdays, breaking my foot (again) as I carried my dialysis fluid from one room to another and spending another year in a cast, the slow demise and inevitable end of my relationship with my girlfriend, feeling constantly cold, motion sickness which kicked in seconds after the car would pull away and made me constantly dry heave, painful oedema (fluid retention) which would seemingly 'drip down' into my lungs at night as if my body was trying to waterboard itself.

To be honest, I know I've forgotten most of it, and I am rather glad I have. I'd became seriously ill in 2005 and I can remember the moment the family doctor told me that he just wanted to 'double-check my kidney function' after a routine blood test, and I remember the epidural needle entering my spine before I was put under for my transplant surgery in 2009, but so much is lost in between. I was in and out of hospital for varying lengths of stay, sometimes after what I thought was a routine check-up (I was instructed to always bring an overnight bag for every appointment), and sometimes as an emergency. I can't give dates, but this pretty much soaked up my thirties.

Here are some 'lowlights':

1)   Low

The nearest I got to a social life while on dialysis was going to hospital appointments, they cluttered and crammed my calendar. A time of particular concern for the doctors was when my blood pressure was so high that it could not even be measured on their industrial looking blood pressure monitor. I was on four different types of medication just to treat this one issue. During a Monday afternoon appointment, a doctor expressed surprise to see me. I asked if I had made a mistake with my appointment time. 'No', he said, 'I didn't think you would survive the weekend. But if I told you that on Friday, then you probably wouldn't have'. He thought he had a measure of my sense of humour. I got the last laugh though; I had to leave that appointment and go for my monthly iron infusion – I collapsed on the way and was immediately admitted for a suspected heart attack.

2)   Lower

You get used to feeling strange and/or painful sensations (migraines, symptoms of a stroke, weird lumps appearing in weird places). Around ten months after I started dialysis, long after my girlfriend had moved out and I was living alone, I was just getting off my sofa to start to prepare my dialysis machine when ... I don't know. I don't know what. I don't know why. I don't know *anything*.

I was in a coma.

The first thing I can remember is waking up to see a painting on a wall that I recognised, but somehow couldn't compute – was it even mine? As I came to, I realised that I was now lying twisted at the top of my stairs – my feet nearer the top of the stairs than my head – and looking at the painting from a previously unviewed angle. Although it would have made sense to call for an ambulance, I reconfigured myself, crawled to my bedroom and managed to phone my mum. 'I think I've been in a coma', I said. And then I stopped remembering the rest of the evening again. I know I was alive the following day though, so I am guessing my mum did something.

3)   Lowest

There are lots of unexpected things about illness and the knock-on effects which one would never even start to consider or imagine. When I first broke my foot, for example, the doctor seemed far more concerned that the inevitable lack of exercise in the near future would turn my slender frame into a bona fide fatty who would need a hoist just to avoid dying of an infected bed sore. That's how doctors think, but it is not necessarily how patients think, and it is certainly not how those pre-plagued by long term chronic health conditions think. Never underestimate the all-consuming power of disease.

In order for peritoneal dialysis to keep your blood spick and span, you need to have as empty a bowel as possible (I don't know why, you just do). However, when you are reduced to drinking just two litres of water a day and prohibited from eating fibrous foods, this is a considerable uphill struggle.

Consequently, among my myriad of meds was a tablet to keep my digestive system running throughout the night. This is, in a healthy body, normally a time your bowels can kick back and relax, however, mine were put to task round-the-clock. On top of that, I was also prescribed a tablet to keep the poo as, *err*, runny as possible. Despite the teamwork of these pills, my digestive system displayed scant regard for getting the 'job' done. Indeed, one X-ray showed I was, and this will come as no surprise to so many people, 'full of shit'.

I could go for several days without a poo, or I could go four times in forty minutes. Either way, what I should have most certainly made a priority is learning how to disengage the dialysis machine, 'unplug' myself from the fluid pump, and take a poo-break.

The lesson came one night in the first few weeks I was on dialysis. I woke with a start as my bowels ground into action and sent a memo to my brain that getting to a toilet was of some urgency. But I was trapped. Connected to a whirring machine with about two metres of slack tube connecting us. There was nothing I could do, as I didn't have time to read the machine's instruction manual. I scanned the room, there was a large black bag which I had used to carry bits of medical equipment. It would have to do. A human poo bag. Hand hygiene was maintained by handfuls and handfuls of alcohol wipes which had become the cornerstone of my hygiene routine.

The bag was disposed of as a matter of urgency the next day in the hazardous waste bin the local council had provided me with. It remains a secret between me, possibly a municipal council worker, and possibly the unluckiest fox in the neighbourhood.

The chasm between shitting in a black polythene bag while squatting on my bedroom floor as a machine as large and as loud as a 1980s dot matrix printer pumped and drained fluid into my abdomen, to the sense of energy ebbing back into my battered body to achieve fully-fledged abso-bloody-lutely amazing levels could not be greater.

In 2009, I was me again. Although technically I was 'me' and some poor '19-year-old male' who was no longer 'him' or in need of his vital organs. The following twelve days post-transplant were not without their ups and downs, but it was not long before I was released into the world.

A world which was in the midst of a pandemic.

Swine flu.

It took me until 2020 to realise quite how little I gave a toss or felt threatened by swine flu. For the first few months post-op in the summer of 2009, I was a walking and talking, festering wound. While I had been in hospital, a skin infection had already found easy passage through my body's patchy immune borders and set up a base camp on the stapled-shut wound they had cut to squish an extra pancreas into me. I had been given the regular prescription pain killers but to no avail. Eventually, my nurses were given the keys to the hospital's cupboard of Class As, and I was given a scrummy opiate lollipop to suck on until the pain subsided. It was a brutal wake-up call to the new immune-supressed state of affairs under which I was now living.

But for some reason, and as I sat there shielded to the hilt from Pandemic Two in 2020, I could not for the life of me think why it didn't occur to me one iota that I could succumb to swine flu. I didn't think to protect myself, nor, for that matter, did any of the doctors I saw.

I can certainly remember hearing news reports about the looming threat, but perhaps the sensory overload of 24-hour doom-mongering news we are all now acclimatised to was yet to gather its current pace.

Transplant surgeons can fall prey to the God complex, so perhaps a transplantée can fall prey to the Lazarus complex? Whatever it was that kept my fears at bay, I wish I had it as the corona pandemic loomed.

Chapter 2
Where did it all go so hopelessly ... right?

A lot can happen from one pandemic to the next. After a quick post-transplant convalesce, it felt like I was being released back into the wild after years of being petted and nurtured in a sanctuary. But was I ready, and what was awaiting me?

Any sense of 'bloke in his thirties in a hetero-normative relationship with a vague semblance of a career' was as dead as the poor donor card-carrying soul who gave me my newfound, abso-bloody-lutely amazing status.

I couldn't claw anything back. The cornerstones of independent living were pulled out from under me: I was no longer able to drive and doubtful I would or could pick up my career where I'd left it. The extended period of my ill health had borne witness to the end of three relatively serious relationships, the latter of which was almost certainly mortally wounded by the battering it took, evoked by my physical and subsequent mental ill health (ranging from hissy fits and tantrums to 'jovial' talk of suicide).

A 'rogue set of blood test results' hardly puts one in the mood for any form of intimacy, and day after day of being poked and prodded by doctors rarely ends with you wanting to pay it forward and poke and prod someone else in the pursuit of carnal pleasure. Having a migraine surely tops having a headache as an 'excuse', and 'I think I am having a stroke' surely tops them both. The truth is, it wasn't long before 'not being in the mood' morphed into 'couldn't even if I wanted to'.

It was not the reason the last of the Organ Failure Relationships fell apart, but it can't have helped. Towards the drawn-out end of that coupling, she moved out for work-related reasons, conveniently just weeks before my dialysis machine moved in. I felt nothing but relief that she only rarely saw me transform into part man, part washing machine as darkness fell every night.

FOR THE (MEDICAL) RECORD

All the way back in 2004 my medical issues amounted to, what felt at the time, 'a little concerning, but hardly life-threatening': a recent eye operation to address a hereditary issue had gone well, but not as well as it perhaps should have, and a misdiagnosed sprained ankle, which had later been determined a shattered foot, had since gone on to calcify and, just about, sort itself out.

I had been working as a news-cum-music journalist and dating a woman who jetted between the UK and the US. In April 2004, I was due to fly to Los Angeles for a six-week, longer-than-usual trip. I had set up interviews with various press contacts in the naïve hope I might be able to scratch myself a living as a music journalist while living under the auspices of my partner.

On the Monday before the Thursday I was due to fly, I had a routine hospital eye appointment so the consultant's good eyes could monitor my slightly dodgy, post-op eyes. All a matter of routine, or so I thought.

'If you get on that plane, you will go blind'.

The words of Doctor Deborah Fleet.

Just another day at the clinic for her, but a life-defining moment for me. She told me I'd need to be referred to, in her exact words, 'the big guns', who were based at Addenbrooke's Hospital in Cambridge.

I left the building in a fog of dismay and panic. Slumped on a bench, I turned my phone on. An unusually elongated flurry of Nokia'd digital burps sounded. That was odd. The only person who was ever that incessant with messaging me was my American girlfriend, and it would have been 3am where she was.

It was my mum. In another building on the same hospital site, my nan had just peacefully passed away. I didn't even know she had been taken to hospital.

Mondays are not supposed to be that great, but *seriously?*

I had always felt that my girlfriend long suspected that I was more in love with the idea of being an LA-based music journalist than I was, well, with *her*. I suspected that she suspected that I found her surplus to this ambition. Her doubting my commitment was a topic which bubbled under every conversation we had at that point.

It came as no surprise that I immediately sensed her *yeah-right-whatever* tone when I called her later that night to tell her my doctors had prohibited me from flying. I had wanted to keep the passing of my nan out of it; it just felt too personal to share at that time. However, when I heard her questioning tone, I rushed in 'andmynanhasdied'. I am not sure she really believed that either, truth be told.

I stopped short of actual fabrication and telling her the cat ate my plane tickets.

I miss LA.

My nan had been living in an elderly people's home, and I had moved into her small house post-eye operation, but before this ocular LA-dream crushing shock. The immediate period after her death saw what we (my mother and I) thought would be a short medical blip to save my eyesight – consisting of further, slightly more-intrusive treatment. It was decided I should continue to stay living in the house for a short while until my eye issue was resolved. That 'short while' ended in November 2010, more than six years later.

That house saw some of the darkest and most depraved sides of my disease and disabilities, not to mention some, presumably indelible, bodily-secreted/leaked stains. It also offered me rent-free sanctuary. I cannot begin to imagine what my life would have been like without that safety net. Had my nan lived longer, the cost of her care would have been paid for by the sale of that property – I try not to dwell on that.

*****

There is no question that life saving transplant surgery will splice into two not only your body but also your life. And while one has to fend off the occasional 'do you think you have the soul of the person who died now in you?' twatty comment, the whole ordeal of both the slow downward spiral of ill-health followed by the supersonic jettison to abso-bloody-lutely amazing that I experienced had a profound effect on me.

During my prolonged absence from the Walking Well and the Working World, my mother had been on a one-woman 'fundraising campaign'. During this time, she had shaken down every purse-string holding employee of the UK government she'd been pointed to by the National Kidney Federation. The result was me being awarded a number of benefits, all of which I was advised I was eligible for by my hospital social worker.

Benefits were directly credited into my account, but at the same time my overheads were surprisingly low, thanks to the altruistic decision by my mother to let me stay in, what was by rights, her pension pot.

From 2004, work was steadily drying up as the internet started its stranglehold on freelance music journalism, and my (then) minor health blips were hardly helping. The more my health spiralled, the more I needed all the financial aid I could get, and the pennies were seemingly just about capable of looking after themselves when I could not eat out, drink out, go on holiday, or even eat 99 per cent of the foods at the supermarket deli end of the shopping spectrum.

There came a point when the only times I ever really left that house was for hospital in-patient stays. When I returned in 2009 post-transplant and convalescence, I checked my bank account. As it appeared, a trickle of benefits (from the pre-Tory-inflicted austerity measures) had formed a puddle of funds which could support my humble life, where my notion of luxury was a latte and a biscotti at the local Caffè Nero.

After the transplant, I was under don't-be-an-idiot and-over-do-it orders from the doctors. Unofficially prescribed to take a year off, I found myself increasingly feeling abso-bloody-lutely amazing, with time on my hands and a modicum of spare change in my pocket.

Even if I had wanted to work, my freelance journalist status had been washed away down the gutter. All my contacts had moved on, and I had no real desire to rejoin the ranks of the 'gutter press' anyway. But my typing fingers were beginning to itch. They sought an outlet and were desperate to defy doctors' orders.

Meanwhile, despite having developed a slight crush on the hospital employee who advised me on my new medications (AKA Pharmacy Girl), I had gone well beyond missing any form of intimacy. It didn't even occur to me. The nerve-battering damage the illness had dealt me seemed like it was just part of this new life, and I was at ease with that. The fact that I was alive and well seemed more than enough. Women and wanking were sectioned off as part of my former life.

Indeed, even before the transplant there were lots of things my body could no longer do thanks to all the damaged bones, tissue, and nerves. Due to the deformed underside of my feet, I was effectively a six-foot Weeble ('Weebles wobble, but they don't fall down'). Unlike a Weeble, however, I did fall down. Quite often, actually.

I'll get to the full tragic tale of my feet later, but even further back in 2002, when the doctor first saw the full extent of my shattered foot bones, he – along with getting a colleague to stand aghast at a deformity they had only seen photos of in medical books – broke the news that I'd never play rugby again. Maybe as a plummy 30-something doctor, he saw that as a life-changing blow, but any chummy bond we might have formed was severed when I told him I had never played rugby anyway. In the interest of good doctor–patient relations, I stopped short of telling him that I considered rugby players to be, in the main, alpha twats.

Away from contact sports, which I'd only ever feigned to play back in my all-boys school days, some things you just get used to not doing anymore, and that list was doubled after being spatchcocked by a team of transplant surgeons. Somehow, none of this seemed to bother me. My life seemed set, simple, and, for the foreseeable future, stable. I had ambitions to get writing again (albeit confined to the blogosphere), a newfound joy of food and drink, and a zeal for life which could be easily and uncomplicatedly lived within my physical constraints.

What I could not have possibly predicted, however, was that 18 months after I was stapled and stitched back together post-transplant, I would be living with my girl-friend. But that's because I also did not predict:

1)   bits of my body which were written-off, did, in fact, still work;

2)   a comment I left on a random blog post would lead to me marrying, albeit many years later, the author of that blog; and

3)   there was more of my life yet to be lived.

*****

If you meet someone on the internet in your mid-thirties, there is always a moment when you have to 'fess up' some-thing from your past (or present) which is not visible on, as it was for us, a MySpace profile photo. Whether you choose the second or third in-real-life date to share the fact that you have 14 children/collect Victorian dolls/have only just come out of prison after a murder charge/webbed toes, it is a moment which plays heavy on your mind.

Imagine the list I had to run through until my conscience was clear enough for her to know exactly what she was getting herself in to.

In 2010, after more than a year of dating, carried out by to-ing and fro-ing between her place and my place, it was crunch time. We had decided to move in together. On the grounds that I had little or no chance of ever finding work in her city, knew no one where she lived, yet had an incredibly supportive network of family, friends and doctors near my (on loan) home without whom I could not have survived, the choice of what to do was obvious.

But apparently not obvious enough.

The real crux, however, was that while my place was in home counties Hertfordshire, UK, her place was in Sweden.

*****

That move to Sweden was ten years before the corona pandemic struck, and while my feet are not as strong as they should be, I did, eventually, metaphorically, find them. In Sweden, my background as a journalist gleaned me work as: a content writer for a lingerie website, for which I wrote in first person about comfort and support; a writer for a publishing house, which produced the kind of inane books only a hipster could love and was, in reality, the vanity project of a psychotic Frenchman; and now, and possibly for good, working for the city university where I specialise in writing about clever people and the clever stuff they do. A job, unlike my other Swedish employment dalliances, I genuinely enjoy.

Tess, or the Swedish Wife as she is known by (my) colleagues, (my) friends, and now even (her) family, knows the soiled tapestry of my 'life once failed', but you can count the number of people who know it in its grimmest detail on one hand, in fact, on one finger – my mother. But we'll get to her later.

It is no secret what I have been through, but the torment my body has endured is not obvious when you look at me. I live under the sword of Damocles, and the Covid 19 virus seemed to me to fray the thread which suspends that sword.

It is not as if I have not succumbed to sniffy colds and feverish flus in the past few years, but none of those bugs has come complete with World Health Organization advice to (at least to my ears), PANIC!

But this is my life now. This is the life I have to maintain and preserve as I embark on this perilous journey and encounter all the pandemics along its pathway.

FOR THE (MEDICAL) RECORD

I look healthy. Healthy enough, anyway.

No one looks at me and quietly ponders with pity, *How does he live like that? How does he sleep/eat/pee?* And as someone with a number of disabilities and significant health issues, I know how very, very fortunate I am to be able to say that.

But here are some things you cannot see: you cannot see that both my feet are acutely deformed with snooker ball-sized bony lumps, so much so I could probably borrow the

Elephant Man's old shoes; you cannot see the transplant scars, so glaringly huge I can jovially pass them off as shark bites; you cannot see the bullet-like wounds where various tubes have been stuck in for months on end or the mysterious hernia-looking bump which I have no clue about, but it doesn't worry the doctors, so it doesn't worry me. You cannot see my wheelchair that I dread I will have to use again. It's currently on loan to a family friend who probably dreaded needing it in the first place. You cannot see any of that, but then, I cannot see you either, at least I cannot see you very well, as my partial-sightedness puts pay to that.

But I look healthy. Healthy enough, anyway. And that's just great, but here's the thing.

For the better part, my outward appearance comes with a sense of 'got away with it', and how very empowering that can feel! But the physical disabilities lurking beneath the scars and lumps are never far from the surface: If I walk too far, my snooker-balled feet are screaming for help using the agonising medium of neuropathic pain, entering a dimly lit shop or restaurant is akin to being in the furthest reaches of a cave with a broken torch, and if I see an oncoming flailing-limbed infant I instinctively and subtly shield myself in fear that a stray fist to the kidney will put me back onto the least desirable of waiting lists. On top of that, I'm permanently weakened by my once-shredded stomach muscles – when I help friends move house, I'm on holding-doors-open and lampshade-carrying duties only.

And it is when those physical ailments expose themselves that my fraudulent healthy exterior comes crashing down and is transformed into a curse, of sorts.

How do you judge the empty-handed man casually

strolling home on a Saturday afternoon while his wife adopts the role of pit pony and lugs two bags of grocery shopping in each hand by his side? What about the seemingly able-bodied passenger who makes a beeline for the last available seat on the bus, a seat reserved for the elderly or disabled? And what about the 40-something who collapses in a heap after miscalculating the steps while exiting a bar at midnight?

Eyes roll, mutters are breathed and disapproving or mocking glances are fired from every angle. By blending in with the 'healthy', I have to blend in with those who display acts of selfishness, laziness, social ineptness and drunkenness.

But putting the *oh, woe is me*-ism aside, online transplant forums are littered with such frustrations, and I'm sure the issue of perceived good health extends well beyond those living off recycled body parts, as grateful as I'm sure we all are.

And it is not just the cynical judging strangers; while our nearests and dearests are still painfully aware of our limitations, it is the extended circles of friends with their 'blimey, last time I saw you, you were in a wheelchair' comments, followed by their 'Wanna trek around Australia for an extreme sports tour?' suggestions that prompt us to reluctantly reel off lingering symptoms and medication side effects.

Once you're off your drip, your dialysis, your chemo, your ... whatever it was that kept you alive long enough for successful treatment to be delivered and the colour has returned to your cheeks, you're perceived once again as a fully functioning adult. Sadly, the reality for many of us is that what has not killed us has made us weaker; the ghosts of past ailments and conditions can still haunt us.

But we walk among you, blending in. We're some of those who trip over, sit on 'reserved for' seats, and walk into lamp posts. Don't judge us.

Chapter 3
The year with ten months

There's been a lot thrown at me over the years – health-wise at least – and 'playing catch' is clearly not my strong point. Friends often seem to double-check themselves when they complain of any ailment which is irking them while in my near vicinity: 'Oh, I know it's not as bad as what you went through'. Everything is relative, I tell them, secretly and safely in the knowledge that it isn't – not even *close*. Fibromyalgia? Yeah, whatever.

I find small mercies where I can, and for 2020, I would say 'not living in China' is all the mercy I was given. While 2020 was quickly written-off as the Worst Year Since Records Began, we seem to forget that a year has 12 months, and if you were living in the West, then January and February were just fine. Corona was little more than a 'whatever, it ain't anywhere near me' news item.

I doubt images of PPE'ed Chinese hospital workers dashing around with patients gasping for their last breaths did little more than provoke a nonchalant 'what's going on over there now, then?' response. In fact, surely ninety per cent of the news footage we ever get from China is of fraught faces partially covered by face masks.

Well, January and February felt fine to me, a bit cold,

dark and wet, but nothing more of note. Indeed, January and February didn't start out any more or less rubbish than January and February 2019, 2018, 2017...

News anchors have somewhat cried wolf when it comes to evoking panic. I doubt the tone they use when they announce an oncoming plague of pandemic potential is any different from the tone they use when rail fares get their annual price hike. Whatever, the news cannot have been that scary, because during the last week of January, we were very much heading in the vague vicinity of China. Not China itself, but in a China-ly direction.

To friends in the UK, a trip to Thailand could smack of a 'holiday of a lifetime', perhaps the kind of prize a family of four might win on a 90s shiny-floor Saturday night quiz show. The Swedes, however, have a rather unique relationship with the country, a relationship that has morphed somewhat over the decades. As it stands, Thailand, to a Swede, is what Benidorm is to a Brit. And the stereotype of a British tourist guzzling down a full, greasy, English breakfast with a can of Stella in Benidorm is the counterpart to the Thai-obsessed Swede. It is alarming how many restaurants in Thailand serve Swedish meatballs.

FOR THE (MEDICAL) RECORD

There's an unusual side-effect to nearly a decade of chronic ill health which only really dawned on me years after my release back into civilisation. And not a side-effect I've ever heard anyone complain about or refer to, or one you'll find in any small print on any medication.

My heavy dose of medically enforced isolation resulted

in a pretty severe case of social and cultural naivety. It only really comes to light when friends or colleagues recall tales of countries they have holidayed to, exotic dishes they have dined on, the gig when whatsherface performed her last ever live show, 'that' stag-do in Prague, 'the' wedding of 2006. People in my peer group seem to have done so much with their lives, and when I am feeling most exposed to these feelings of missed-outness, it dawns on me that they are often recollecting memories from their thirties: a period of my life peppered, then saturated with incapacity, inability, and mind fog-induced indifference to the world around me.

It wasn't as if this decade was a total loss for me, I did my best to max out what my body would allow me to do, as and when my body would allow me to do it. In fact, I once hobbled around Slovenia on crutches and sold a travel piece to a tourist trade magazine specialising in over-60s tours. However, it wasn't long into my thirties that my body could do absolutely zilch-all.

During my dialysis days, I had to spend every night at home; I had to be in bed by 10pm to ensure my dialysis could complete all its cycles before my cat wanted his breakfast. In regard to my diet, I suspect even the most devout monk would cast off his cassock and bid a blasphemous farewell to his lord if he got to the monastery and saw a menu as bleak as the one I had forced upon me.

So while my friends were enjoying their steady income, pre-kid, budget airline jet-set lives, I was medically restrained. I could not eat out, go out or stay out. My peers now seem to know what they like based on experiences of trial and error. The simple economic principle of opportunity cost means that I have not had the time, opportunity or budget to experience or explore.

So, even now, as I ebb ever further towards my fifties, I am still figuring out what floats my boat and tickles my fancy. I don't know what I like, because there is a good chance I have never tried it before.

I only went on a handful of travels and holidays between the ages of 20 and 40. I am doing my best to catch up, but I don't appreciate raised eyebrows and looked down noses when I excitedly try a new food for the first time or choose to go to Spain ... or Thailand.

*****

We were more than aware that we were ebbing towards the corona hotspots as we flew. After we landed, we queued at passport control surrounded by pasty western faces and masked-to-the-hilt Chinese tourists, the latter of which were to-ing and fro-ing as part of their new year celebrations.

From cleaner to cabin crew, and co-pilots to coach driver, we didn't see any member of staff at the airport or in the airport's general vicinity who was not wearing a mask. I would say it brought the pandemic home, but it felt more like we were 'going back to its place'.

Still, the bumpier the roads got as we drove away from the airport, the less corona-y everything seemed to be. At the time, Thailand had the most cases outside of China, although all the cases they did have were Chinese tourists – which passport control queues were they in? An exception was a Thai person who had just flown in from the corona epicentre, Wuhan. The fact that we were in a relatively remote resort seemed to provide an ample buffer zone for our peace of mind.

I wouldn't necessarily regard myself as a tropical beach kind of holidaymaker, but years of living with disabilities have made me and the bargain end of the Tropics somewhat comfortable deckchair-fellows. So many of my peers can ski, trek, dive with sharks (although, as I said, my scars suggest I tried this once and have all the evidence to justify I should never do it again); the rest have kids and seem duty-bound to spend their much-needed time off work trailing around gawdy overpriced theme parks.

Meanwhile, I am advised by my foot specialist against walking on uneven surfaces. That rules out everything from quaint cobbled streets to forest floors to theme parks littered with discarded Disney-themed detritus.

The medication I take makes me prone to skin cancer, something which rules out the dry scorch of the peak-season Mediterranean sun. Thailand and thereabouts, at least at the time we travel, is both comfortably warm and blissfully overcast with abundant cloud cover. Either way, the first thing I do every morning when I am in such a climate is stand naked in the bathroom and slather on factor 50 suntan lotion, covering everything from toes, testicles and temples – if I catch a glimpse of myself in the mirror, I look like a six-foot albino skid mark.

My slender frame and deformed feet lend me the physique of a golf club, but I do rather enjoy the 'I walk among you' thrill I can get when no one knows quite what a physical wreck I am.

Indeed, I remember my first ever weekend trip to Sweden. Tess (not yet the Swedish Wife) had gone to work, and I was free to plod the evenly-paved streets of the city of Malmö on my tod. I went to a café, ordered a latte, and sat in the best people-watching corner I could find. I knew no one else in the city other than Tess, and for the first time for a very long time, it occurred to me that no one could tell how disabled I am. I was not in a wheelchair, there were no crutches lying by my side on the floor which I had to constantly shift to avoid tripping up a pensioner, no one had to guide me in and help me to sit down, and there was no chance I may have ignored anyone by accident – which I so often do due to my partial eyesight. It was utterly liberating. I dwelled on that. I became overwhelmed with emotion about how far I had come in such a short period of time. I started to tear up a little. Then I was the weird bloke sitting by himself discreetly sobbing in the corner. There were raised eyebrows. Oh well, back to square one!

*****

In my day-to-day life, I don't feel like I get dressed every morning, I feel like I am putting on a disguise. And I've gotten pretty good at mastering my camouflage. Over the years, I have figured out what best hides my foot deformities and my new kidney which freakishly protrudes from my lower abdomen.

Dressing for sunny climes, however, is when this disguise can so easily fall away. All the evidence suggests that no one really cares what they look like as they shuffle around the breakfast buffet in their flip-flops, with tit fat and beer belly lolloping and leaking out over the trays of fruit platters, sausages and bacon. I obviously cannot wear jeans (which I normally wear with a turn-up, as the double-fabric thickness of it subtly shields my bulbous feet), as then I'd be adding sweat-induced nappy rash to my list of woes.

Nor can I wear my regulation orthopaedic boots, which have a soupçon of 'army surplus' about them, that I utilise whenever I am embarking on uncharted ground and all the surfaces that could present themselves. A partially covered veranda in Thailand is no place to look like you are a wannabe booted-up militiaman. Also, under no circumstances can I ever walk barefoot. From the moment I step out of bed, my feet are protected by either orthopaedic house slippers, orthopaedic insoles, or the aforementioned orthopaedic clumpy boots.

Before my travels, my orthotics specialist had made me some, what I offensively call 'spaz sandals'. On presenting them to me, she informed me that I was never ever ever to wear them unless I was also wearing socks. Great. Socks and sandals. As if I didn't feel self-conscious enough as it was.

The very real fear is that if one of my deformities was to rub against the fabric of the sandal, a blister could turn to an infection within days, leading to the very real possibility of amputation. When it comes to socks and sandals, pride cannot come before a fall if the reason you fall is that you only have one foot to stand on.

I opted for sneakers with orthotic insoles. I try to keep as much of my body as covered as possible, so linen trousers instead of shorts, and a linen shirt instead of a t-shirt. A baseball cap only shades the face, but a Panama hat shades both the face and the neck, so that is what I plump for. The Swedish Wife tells me that I look more like I am going on an empire-building exercise rather than a holiday.

Add all that to the fact that it is more often the case that I am the only British person around, so while I might look and sound like a posh English twat to the eyes and ears of Europe's sun-seekers, I don't feel paranoid that people are double-taking my lumps, bumps and scars and wondering if I am a taking a break from my career as a circus freak.

(I appreciate that is probably not what they would think anyway, but in my head, they are, and I am the one who has to live in my head.)

FOR THE (MEDICAL) RECORD

They were somewhat unlikely surrounds for my mind to meander into a psychotic, violent fantasy; eating breakfast, as I was, in the luxurious grounds of a Southeast Asian hotel – proper holiday of a lifetime type stuff, if you will.

I was sitting on an open air, shaded veranda with monstrous fans gently encouraging a cooling breeze through linen drapes to counter the rising tropical daytime climes.

I should have been gazing upon the sweeping, manicured lawns as they flowed seamlessly into the white sands of the resort's hidden beach. But I wasn't. What I actually was doing was imagining my thumbs crushing the windpipe of the man who sat two tables away.

My violent fantasy had omitted the detail of how my ten-stone, disabled body had managed to manoeuvre itself into such a position, what with him being a twenty-something, bronzed, athletic, muscled type, or indeed, why his apparent gym bunny breakfast companion had done nothing to aid him.

His crime? Well, it could be that he had used the hotel's unfathomable toaster with some aplomb, which had put me on my back foot (why is it only ever me who suffers from breakfast buffet stress?). But no, it was his t-shirt which tipped me into such ire. It read,

'Life Begins Outside Your Comfort Zone'.

'FUCK YOU', my inner monologue raged.

The slogan was complemented by an extreme sport graphic of, what I'm going to refer to as a 'dude', doing something 'extreme' and 'sporty' on the crest of a wave.

Of course the kneejerk reaction is to contemplate the logic – if you're happy doing it, then it isn't really outside of your comfort zone. I think what he was actually trying to convey was that he is someone who likes throwing himself off cliffs, or whatever, and the garment was worn with the intention that the person noting the wording would be impressed.

My counter t-shirt might read: 'Extreme Sports Are of Little or No Interest to Me'.

Besides all that, is that what 'comfort zones' are really about? I normally hear them in the contexts of public speaking, job interviews, stage performances. Maybe the image on his t-shirt should have depicted an empty rostrum and an awaiting audience, naked bar their socks.

As my fantasy ensued and he gurgled pleas for me to stop, I started to consider when I have been the furthest outside of my comfort zone.

Having been temporarily blind, spent around two years with both feet in casts, been on kidney dialysis, and had a double organ transplant, I've got my fair share to choose from.

Here's just one:

The insertion of the peritoneal dialysis tube into the peritoneal cavity was not as routine 'as advertised'. After the tube was first inserted, I started dialysis only for most of the blood cleansing fluid to stay in my gut. I returned to the hospital after a few days looking like I was 15 months pregnant, and an emergency decision was made to insert a new tube.

I was given a local anaesthetic and a strong sedative, which promptly knocked me out. A general anaesthetic was not required for such a simple and quick procedure, I was assured.

However, I woke up with a surgeon seemingly wrist-deep in my guts. 'I'm AWAKE', I pleaded. 'Almost done', he insisted. I could now feel the pain as the anaesthetic wore off.

The reality of the situation engulfed me. I was awake, ably conversing with a man who was fumbling around with my innards. To add insult to injury, I had not changed into a hospital gown and the fluid which had inflated me had now leaked out onto the bed. I was having this conversation while effectively lying in five litres of my own piss, which was slowly soaking into my pulled down jeans and rolled up jumper.

All things considered, I was outside of my comfort zone, and at no point did I think, *life is beginning*.

Life, in fact, felt very much like it was drawing to a close.

Take that, surf dude.

But then, as my imagined death grip on his throat loosened and his sobbing partner composed herself, something did occur to me. After almost a decade of ill health, I was now sitting in a beautiful spa retreat, healthy and happy.

Maybe those excursions outside of my comfort zone were where a life was beginning after all, or, at the very least, restarting.

Still a fucking stupid t-shirt, mind.

*****

So, on we go with our holiday. We kept ourselves to ourselves with mild-mannered sightseeing and swimming in pools and seas, but occasionally I found myself tuning into BBC radio and hearing the latest reports as the corona pandemic slipped on its executioner's mask and strode to the global gallows.

The death count was still low and, as far as the collective ethnocentric eyes of the West was concerned, still China's problem. I probably would not have been so attentive to the news if I was still in northern Europe and not in China's apparent playground. I did, if we passed a pharmacy, pop in and check to see if they had any alcohol gel, having since started to dabble with the stuff. They had always sold out.

Up until this point, I had never so much as sniffed alcohol gel in my life, not even for recreational use, but Tess had two small bottles which came with some travel packs we'd been given and only hung on to as they contained little toothbrushes which we used on the flight over. The little bottles of gel were becoming increasingly treasured.

Things changed for me when Tess said she had found some 'disabled-friendly jungle' we could explore. The only way to get there would be to go on an 'adventure day' during which we would be driven to various markets and temples before Thailand's answer to a gondola boat trip into the jungle. Nothing makes me shudder quite like the words 'adventure day', but Tess was keen, and she'd found the most Adrian-friendly tour available.

We had no idea what to expect, but I think we were both a little taken aback when we realised that the day would only be us, a driver, and a guide. That's a little too much conversational pressure for the likes of us; I am the chatty one, but I tend to look for one iota of common ground to launch into chat and knew I'd struggle to find a shred to talk about with two people who like trekking through itchy, bite-y and spiky bits of nature. But it was too late to back out without losing a deposit, so we met with them bright and early and before we had too much time to discuss the pros and cons, or rather the cons and cons, of endless awkward social interactions.

The driver was waiting for us outside the SUV which would be our transport until we got to the boat. The guide was a fresh-faced young Thai, the driver was ... not. He looked like Death warmed up, or was that, he looked like he was fresh from Death's deep freeze. It was hard to tell; he was both sweating and shivering in equal measure. And coughing. He coughed a lot.

Bollocks.

He wore a face mask, but he only raised it from his chin to cover his nose and mouth after he started to splutter and sneeze; he would simultaneously roll down the window as he did so. Then wind it back up the moment the coughing eased. The car had air conditioning; it was hard not to imagine the swirling particles of snot that were being blasted around us, in us.

The guide explained that it was common for locals to

display such symptoms when the start of the rainy season prompted such a respiratory response. I've yet to credit that theory with a cursory google. Effectively we were trapped in an airtight car with him for around five hours, with whatever he was pumping out of his lungs with the erratic accuracy of a sawn-off shotgun. A snotgun.

At one point he pulled over to buy, and then glug down in one gulp, a can of Red Bull. He could not have been any more evidently sick if he was wrapped in a blanket and nursing a cup of Lemsip.

It's hard to truly appreciate breath-taking views when you think you might be contracting a breath-taking virus while you take in the vista. It could have been a trip of a lifetime if only I could have removed the thought from the back of my mind that this might be the last trip I ever take in my lifetime.

My logical conclusion, however, was not that he might be suffering from the dreaded covidz – that just seemed so unlikely at the time, but rather that if we were to contract any form of fever from him, it would be nigh-on impossible to navigate our way back through Bangkok airport, where we knew temperature checks were now in place.

We felt like jungle fever ticking time bombs upon our return to our hotel room.

Fortunately, we never detonated.

*****

We were now coming towards the end of the holiday and I-just-wanna-get-back levels of anxiety were rising fast. As the roads towards the airport got smoother and smoother, evidence of the encroaching pandemic increased. And that evidence was infinitely more compelling than the last time we travelled these roads, just two weeks earlier.

One domestic flight later, and we were in Bangkok, where images I had only ever seen on the telly were dramatically unfolding in front of us. Now, more than half the people we saw were wearing face masks – the returning Chinese tourists with their masks snuggly fitted. Meanwhile, the European mob mainly wore theirs under their chins while they munched on Burger King meals; others had them covering just their mouths, just their noses, and, for some children, only their ears.

Clearly Europeans were newbies when it came to a pandemic.

We returned to Sweden on February 9th, where there had now been one reported case. We were back at ease watching the pandemic unfold from the safety of our own home.

Not long after, however, Europe was in the embryonic stages of oblivion and the sub-conscious fear in my brain was rising to the surface. Old people seemed to be the virus's host/victim of choice, and for some inexplicable and illogical reason, in my brain, that meant that old people were the most likely to have it.

On March 5th, I went to a classical concert with a friend after his mother bailed last minute and left him with a spare ticket. We sat among a sea of grey-haired and frail-looking concert goers, and I had never felt so threatened. We went on to a crowded wine bar. On March 11th, I was in a cellar comedy club watching a Romanian comedian: 'If you don't have it yet, you've almost certainly got it now', he joked.

The following day, as more and more cases were reported in Sweden, I made an executive decision to work from home. As I packed up my laptop, my boss came to my desk. Well aware of my vulnerability, she ratified my decision: 'Get yourself home' was the order.

That was March 12th. At around 11am, I cycled home through the city as a storm gathered. My ride home took me past a usually placid seafront. The waters stirred. The sign with the meal deal of the day outside the 7 Eleven had been blown over. The skies were blackening. It quite genuinely felt like a penultimate scene from a Netflix season 1 finale.

The Corona Saga had begun.

Chapter 4
Yeah, like I didn't see that coming

It's not every day that a member of middle management walks up to your desk mid-morning to announce that she and a cabal of other managers have agreed that, due to an oncoming plague from the east and in fear I might succumb to said plague, I should probably work from home for the foreseeable future. In fact, the more I think about it, the more I convince myself that this is indeed the first time 'my possible imminent death' had ever been discussed in the workplace (at least to my knowledge).

Which begged the question, where was this overwhelming sense of déjà vu coming from?

The truth is, that over the course of my ill-health, along with the physical scars, my psyche has taken a bit of a bashing. I am sure I have early childhood memories of being an optimist, and I am sure I was blessed with a carefree nature throughout my teens and then beyond. But now I live with a curse, a sixth sense. A sense I never wanted, but one I was gifted with all the same – the gift of a Cynical Sixth Sense.

Not much of a gift really, as an extra sense is so often perceived as being. I can't 'see dead people', in fact the only dead person I can really picture is myself. Not really a gift you want to be given at all, and a gift I can't take back and exchange for a better sense, like, I don't know, common sense.

I am just too used to life-defining moments of 'oh, for fuck's sake, what *now*?'.

I never used to expect the worst, but the worst kept happening all the same: *Oh look, now I am in a wheelchair. Whatever,* 'your heart is not strong enough to undergo surgery, so we're going to have to take you off the transplant waiting list'... *boring,* or 'looks like we'll need to circumcise you'... I'm sorry, *what? Pfft,* 'Okay, just get on it with it'.

Why would I not return from a holiday in the Tropics only to find out that Judgement Day had been added to this year's calendar? And my judgement was set to come in the form of a Covid-positive test result.

*****

It was probably in early 1999 when I could last count my senses on just one hand, although even then my sense of touch was fast depleting after the hammering my fingertips had gotten from constant blood test lancet punctures.

I had sprained or twisted my left ankle. I'm not even sure how it happened. All I remember is it hurting and me hobbling. I did all the tokenistic lazing around with my foot elevated and resting on a pack of frozen peas that any matronly nurse could reasonably expect of a bloke in his late twenties to do.

The swelling was lingering, and I'd tried to squish and squash the lump which had flared up on the side of my foot, but it was neither squishy nor squashy, it just felt like solid bone.

'It can feel like solid bone', the locum doctor confirmed after giving it a medically certified squish and squash himself. I had been prompted by my this-cannot-be-right paranoia/hypochondria to visit my village doctor's surgery. He ordered me off for an X-ray just to be on the safe side, and days later it was confirmed that indeed, there were no breaks to be seen.

I'm not sure who I thought I was to question an X-ray machine, but I did. That X-ray was wrong, I just knew it. I felt it, quite literally, in my bones. The embryonic stages of my new sense were coming into being.

Even so, off I hobbled. And over 20 years later that hobble and that solid bony lump remain. The doctor had been right, the X-ray machine had been right, my foot was not broken – it was completely shattered.

Months after that first visit I had returned to the local surgery and presented the same lump to a different doctor. He sent me off to a bigger, better, shinier X-ray machine, and it was then that the shattered foot was diagnosed, although in 'medical speak' it is actually referred to as a Lisfranc fracture. I was told such an injury had resulted in hundreds of micro fractures which a common or garden X-ray machine was not capable of detecting.

But not to worry (yeah, right), the bones had calcified and as long as I didn't do any excessive weight-bearing exercise, I should be fine. 'It might get a little arthritic in 30 years', the man with my X-rays optimistically warned me. The same man who wrongly assumed I might be a rugby player. He added that this was a prevalent injury among Crimean War calvary men who had been blasted off their horses and got a foot caught in a stirrup; I would be lying if I said I didn't think that sounded like quite a sexy injury to live with.

In 2004, and five years later ...

The little bony lump was now a slightly bigger bony lump, and the hobble was now a bona fide limp. I was back at the village surgery with a very hurty foot in the company of a very worried looking practice nurse. I knew back in 1999 that the doctors were wrong, and I had been proved right. I wasn't going to make the same mistake again.

That Cynical Sixth Sense was now as much a part of me as my protruding lump. Something was 'afoot'.

Sent directly to hospital, I was given a thorough scanning and a new, far more sinister diagnosis was given: a neurological progressive degeneration foot disorder.

Check this out for part of the condition's Wiki entry: 'If this pathological process continues unchecked, it can result in joint deformity, ulceration and/or superinfection, loss of function, and in the worst-case scenario, amputation or death.'

Superinfection? Death? Fucking *death*? Who dies of a sprained ankle?! I had already gotten to the joint deformity stage.

The nurse who fitted me into a plastic boot to stem the damage was in jovial and reassuring form. She called it a 'Beckham boot' because all she really knew about me was my name, gender, and the fact that I was (now) in my thirties, ergo I must like football; she also knew that David Beckham had recently had to wear a similar boot after buggering up his foot. It was assumed I was a footie fan. I let it slide.

My medical records were updated to include the Victor Hugoian description of 'acutely deformed', and I was sent on my way. 'You can drive home, but then that's it. You need to rest', the nurse nonchalantly informed me.

I hadn't known what to expect when I drove to the hospital that day. But I knew she was only telling me not to drive until my foot was healed. Upon my return, I parked up outside my house, took my newly assigned NHS crutches from the back seat and hobbled in. That niggling Cynical Sixth Sense had grown in certainty and was telling me that I would probably never drive again. There was no real reason to think that but think it I did – it was more than a niggle, it was more than a hunch. I just *knew* it. And I have never been back behind the wheel since.

Life was increasingly justifying my worst fears with reality.

I had been using my car less and less anyway. Once a hack for hire, who daily had to dash off to doorstep or stalk the next poor victim the tabloid media had in its crosshairs, I was now slowly morphing into a London-based music journalist and largely getting around by train and tube.

On that era-defining morning, everything changed. I was now forced to work from home ... forced to try to work from home, at least. My career and my health were in an apparent intertwined downward spiral. When you are just a voice on a phone, or the sender of an email, you can get away with appearing fully functional, but the moment the conversation turned to 'Can you just get to...?', the job was over. Then, within months, all the jobs were over.

I was becoming a disabled person. It's a slippery slope and – particularly when you can't grip with your deformed foot – it's a difficult slope to climb back up.

While I didn't quite fit the mould, the assumption was – during casual conversations at least – that this was some form of sport-related injury. The assumption was often backed up with the reassurance that bones heal in about six weeks. I just couldn't bring myself to explain to all and sundry that this injury would take at least a year to heal.

Months into treatment, I felt a twinge in my other foot. That twinge prodded my Cynical Sixth Sense back into action: this was bad. I cautiously limped straight to the doctor. There was nothing visible this time, nothing to poke, nothing to prod, nothing to ponder on, nothing – as the doctor explained – to worry about.

And they were wrong again. Another victory for that Cynical Sixth Sense.

Within weeks the right foot had grown a matching bony lump. My feet were out of control, and my local GP could not handle this. My local hospital could not handle this. I, and my increasingly deforming feet were sent to a King's College Hospital in London, which has its very own department for the treatment of wonky feet.

Life as I had known it was coming to a close.

Nothing is quite as soul destroying as a doctor taking one look at you, excusing himself, only to return moments later with a camera. That doctor then called a colleague over to debate the freakshow before them. As he happily snapped away for either research or, well, the mind boggles, reasons, they both concluded this problem was above their pay grade.

Soon, other colleagues gathered to gawk, but this time, salvation had arrived, the head honcho, the best professor of feet in town. I didn't know it then, but this man was to go on to save my life – feet first.

Professor Mike Edmonds had a certain nervous energy akin to a British Woody Allen; while mature enough in years, he wore a lab coat like he had borrowed it from his dad and was playing dress-up. What, however, was abundantly clear, was that he had the respect of his department, his peers, and as I now understand, leading foot nerds from around the world. Indeed, years later in a Swedish foot clinic, I dropped his name into conversation only to be met with looks I imagine were not dissimilar to those that some are reserving for the Second Coming.

His team took one look at the boot I had been fitted with and threw it away. I was given the Nike Air Jordan equivalent of medical boots for one foot, and the most recently deformed foot was put in a cast.

That slippery slope into disability was now a lot more slippery.

No casual conversationalist ever assumed it was a football injury again. I told people I was in the SAS and had broken both feet in a parachute accident. Clearly a lie, and clearly the most diplomatic way of telling them to 'fuck off'. I wasn't in the mood for questions or giving answers. I started to dread bumping into people I knew who had seen me in the cast months beforehand; an internal war waged between my gregarious nature and my face-saving desire to retreat into reclusiveness.

As I was treated, I was also investigated, and it wasn't long until it was concluded that my bones were not quite as strong as they should be, at least in my feet and lower legs. I was about a year into treatment when the professor suggested I try a drug which had hitherto only been used on the nan/granddad generation. It was an injection I was to self-administer, and while I was on the drug I was under some very watchful eyes.

I don't know how long it was after I started that medica-

tion, but I know it was the week that my local general practitioner doctor had first spotted my rogue kidney blood
test results. Predictably, I had been on a bit of a downer
ever since hearing the news that my kidneys were not pulling their weight. I now had to go back to the GP to repeat
the blood test the following week ('just drink lots of water
before the test – I'm sure it'll be fine', he told me, even
though my Cynical Sixth Sense was screaming the opposite). It was also the week I was due to have a routine appointment with Professor Edmonds.

I had gone out on a Sunday afternoon stroll/hobble to
clear my head when my phone rang. It was the professor.
'Do you think you could come in a little earlier than your
Tuesday appointment?' he asked.

I assumed this was just an admin thing, although it
did seem a little odd that he was calling, apparently from
home, on a Sunday afternoon. I could hear someone in the
background making cooking noises. I suggested Monday.

'How about you come in now?' he said, with a warm reassuring tone which I heard as 'get down here *as soon as
possible.*'

It turned out that the professor had also noted I had
flunked a kidney test, and he was quite clearly panicking
that this might be due to the drug I was regularly sticking
myself with under his direction.

A week as an inpatient ensued, where I had to monitor
every drop of fluid I consumed and lug around a sloshing
bucket of piss I had to empty that fluid into. Within days,
my kidney function returned to normal, and the relief on
the professor's face was palpable. He told me that a note
would be made regarding that drug and its use on younger generations. I was discharged, and we all went on our

merry little ways.

You could probably rearrange the letters which make up his qualifications after that professor's name and complete the alphabet ... twice, but that's no match for my Cynical Sixth Sense. I knew the trajectory of my underlying health condition, and I knew I still needed to do another – now delayed – kidney blood test for my local doctor.

In 1989, I got an F grade for my Graphic Communication high school exam. I had never failed a test so badly before, or since. Until now.

My kidneys were not fine – not at all. Whatever blip had suggested they were when I was an inpatient was quickly disregarded. All of a sudden, my feet, which apparently could lead to my death, were the least of my woes. My creatinine levels – used to monitor kidney function – were on the up, my wee was the colour of budget supermarket tropical flavoured fizzy pop (and smelt about as bad), and my poo sample looked like something an Asphalt sales rep carried around in a briefcase.

I was admitted to a kidney ward, in the same London hospital that housed the wonky foot department, where I was to share a room with a ... I'm not sure, it looked dead. It had visitors though, and they would talk to it as if it were still alive and bring it things which corpses have no need for, like magazines.

That 'corpse' was actually a particularly friendly man, who I, during the fleetingly brief moments when we were both lucid and awake at the same time, would exchange hospital small talk, which nimbly skirted around the obvious *what-the-hell-is-wrong-with-you?* line of questioning.

He had greasy curls plastered into his hollowed cheeks, his skin was mottled and grey and his eyes were too far back in his skull for me to gauge, when he was not talking, whether he was conscious or not. Our beds faced each other, about four metres apart, but I could smell his distinct yet unfathomable odour from where I lay.

Was this my future? The Ghost of Christmas You're Fucked. I don't know what happened to him. I can't remember much about him other than the fact that he didn't like hospital yogurt and I didn't like hospital ham, so we'd do swapsies at lunchtime. It was seeing him, almost like a reflection, and knowing that we were deemed worthy of the same level of care, that made me understand quite how sick I was.

The hospital was hours away from where I lived, and despite my mum and my friends making the journey when they could, I had never felt so alone.

There were times when the curtains for the windows which divided the room from the ward corridor were swished closed, just randomly it seemed. Then the door to our room would be gently and discreetly closed. There'd be a silence. The bleeps and the bloops of the machines were still audible, the moans and the groans, while now dampened by the closed doors, were still ever present, but there was something different marked by a slowing down of commotion. Then, the sound of shuffling nurses' scrubs performing some rehearsed movements from the corridor. Then silence again.

Perhaps 20 minutes would go by, sometimes longer. Somewhere in a side room, news was being broken, and then the silence was broken, too. The sound of mournful howls, and weeping. Sometimes, perhaps even more tragically, nothing. No one to break news to, nothing but the resumption of the everyday cacophony of ward life. A ward with a freshly made bed for a new in-patient. Out with the old …

This was purgatory, or at the very least, the last stop before the Final Destination.

Maybe it's a smidge of PTSD, but I don't really remember much about that time. I know my mum's eyebrows fell out with the stress; something she likes to remind me about to this very day – something she blames me for. They stabilised me enough to discharge me, but the Cynical Sixth Sense was in overdrive.

I was now a regular attendee at the kidney clinic, where every visit would reveal the news of the ever-decreasing function of my kidneys. The concepts of 'dialysis' and 'transplant' were now just 'matters of time' rather than 'worst case scenarios'.

One day, I was asked,

'Would you like a pancreas as well as a kidney?'.

It was a question delivered with the same nonchalance of a McDonald's drive-thru attendant asking me if I wanted 'fries with that'. And in keeping with the tone, and in the manner of someone 'super-sizing' their burger order, I recall my response being 'why not?'.

The consultant looked at his computer screen, clearly clocked my home counties Hertfordshire address, and then remarked 'people with that postcode tend to survive this'. I was so unaware of my privilege at that time that I left the room more baffled by that remark than I was traumatised by this momentous decision I had just made. After all, for me to have a double organ transplant, someone who was living a healthy life at that very moment, would have to die.

And that someone turned out to be a 19-year-old male,

so perhaps at the time I made that decision he was just a 15-year-old teenager, with copies of *Fast Bikes* magazine strewn across his bedroom floor and a motorbike-shaped piggy bank on a shelf that he was using to save up for when he was old enough to get his provisional licence and his first bike.

This was about two years after my initial meeting with Professor Edmonds, and I was now able to hobble around with the aid of orthotics, which supported the backs of my lower legs. I had become a regular at his clinic, and he had given me both his home and mobile phone numbers. The woman who had been making the cooking noises in the background when he called that Sunday afternoon was his wife, and she now knew me by my first name. On the one occasion I had to call him at home, she heard my name and responded with immediate recognition.

He had been with me every limping step of the way. Above and beyond the call of duty, determined to get me back on my feet. He'd joke around with my mum and re-membered things I had said in idle chat while he inspected my lumps, from three conversations prior. I thought he saw in me something special, that we had bonded, but then I spoke to other patients he had treated. I wasn't spe-cial at all. *He* was.

The King's College Hospital chapter was coming to a close. It was agreed that after the dialysis tube was insert-ed into me, my care would be transferred to the hospital in Cambridge, much nearer to where I lived, and also where the 'big guns' who were continuing their battle to save my eyesight were based. The one-stop shop for all my health requirements.

It was a period of time when both my physical and mental health had been battered beyond recognition. When an inkling of fear that something could go wrong had been replaced with the cynical 'knowledge' that it most certainly will go wrong.

I recall being driven to my mother's house, where I was increasingly seeking solace and sanctuary whenever I could. I had just been delivered more brutal news about my health status. 'We'll just get home, and you can rest. The day cannot get any worse now', my mum said, with her one-day-at-a-time positive mentality. I told her not to say that, jokingly scolding her that she might jinx the day.

Later that evening, I was urgently admitted into hospital.

And that was the mentality I brought with me as we collectively succumbed to the pandemic. I've not read a science textbook since I was fifteen, so my knowledge has never been called upon as part of a Prime Minister briefing in either Sweden or the UK, but my Cynical Sixth Sense had known better than that first doctor who misdiagnosed my swollen foot, and I sure wasn't buying into any notion that we would be out of this pandemic by Easter 2020, or indeed – as it was first suggested – that it might not wash up on our shores.

I was doomed, and there was nothing anyone could say or do to persuade me otherwise.

*****

As for Professor Edmonds, I actually bumped into him in Sweden in 2017 when he was visiting the university where I now work. I excitedly bounded up to him as if he was my 'O Captain! My Captain!' English teacher and I his star pupil. I rattled off some snippets of my medical history in a bid to spark his memory. I could see it slowly dawn on him who I was. 'Oh, do pass on my regards to your mother', he said, before he dashed off.

And as for the man in the bed opposite, my Ghost of Christmas You're Fucked, I hope beyond hope he is well. I hope he is somewhere in London writing a book about the time he was ill. Maybe he has mentioned the man who looked as near to a corpse as he could imagine it is possible to be. The man with greasy curls plastered into his hollowed cheeks, his skin mottled and grey, and his eyes too far back in his skull for him to gauge – when he was not talking – whether he was conscious or not. The guy in the bed opposite, his distinct yet unfathomable odour putting him off his double-ham sandwich. The guy that was me.

Chapter 5
Headlines, timelines, and flatlines

Cynical Sixth Sense aside, what became fast apparent, as the virus took flight, was that nothing brings out my inner self-protective, psychotic nature quite like the embryonic stages of the death of civilisation.

Truth be told, I've never been much of a risk taker; for as long as I can recall, I've taken a step back and allowed either a brother, a friend or a lover to swim as far as 'that' buoy, take a puff on 'that' pipe, stick 'that' up 'there'.

That self-protective nature of mine went into stellar hyper-overdrive the moment I regained consciousness after that ten-hour-plus transplant surgery. The second-hand offal nestled in quickly, with no real snags having me as their new landlord, and I am certainly never planning to terminate their lease.

Before all this pandemic nonsense, quite how psychotic my self-protectionism is had never really been put to task. If you ever ask me whether there is anyone in the world I'd 'take a bullet for', then you'll either be offended or lied to. The truth is, absolutely no one. A rather selfish attitude perhaps – bearing in mind what so many people have done for me over the years – but I think my nearest and dearest have come to expect nothing less. They know how seriously I take my own welfare.

Prior to this pandemic, that mentality would play out in its most extreme form when my wife and I watched any variety of post-apocalyptic zombie television series. We would bark orders at the telly in a non-committal bid to save the characters from their predictable torn-sinew-from-gristle dooms.

What dawned on me faster than the dead, however, was how often our futile, life-saving guidance would be the polar opposite to one another's. How we would navigate such a scenario led to a mutual agreement of 'when the zombie-shit hits the doomsday-fan, there is no bloody way I am sticking with you' agreement. As threats to a relationship go, this was unlikely to be troubling any marriage counsellor any time soon.

Unlikely.

And there we were, in the eye of the corona shitstorm. A vaccine would be 'with us within the year', or 'highly likely to never appear', depending on which boff in a lab coat you chose to believe. Either way, where have I heard the line 'It all started when scientists raced to find a vaccine to save humankind from a lethal virus'? How many B-movie scriptwriters have had to lazily fall back on that tired old trope? How else has a zombie apocalypse ever even started?

Fact was fast catching up with fiction, and the zombie dilemma that had only jovially 'plagued' our relationship was coming to a very real and rotten/decomposing head. The actual Apocalypse Reality Show was just a few episodes in, and already I could see her survival tactics were sealing our mutual fates.

Sweden was the 'safe farmhouse' in this scenario, but I

wanted to flee to the 'community in the compound' – more commonly known as 'my mum's house in the UK'.

Tess was towing the Swedish nonchalant line, which amounted to little more than 'try not to sneeze in someone else's face', while I was being aurally drip-fed BBC reports of an imminent lockdown. While scenes of Italian hospitals were making the average Brit shunt their plate of spaghetti bolognaise to one side, the Swedes were still packing their skis and heading into the eye of Europe's epidemic epicentre in northern Italy.

The UK was clearly my sanctuary and my best chance of survival. The world seemed to be going into mutually agreed panic stations, apart from Sweden, a country that would soon be the global odd one out.

Tess eventually relented, albeit partially. It was an approval begrudgingly borne from my UK-media-fuelled fear. If needs-must, she would herself deliver me from evil via the means of a road trip. A road trip that would take us through Denmark, The Netherlands, Belgium and France – a proposal which was starting to feel ever so slightly *Mad Max*-y.

Leaving the 'Swedish farmhouse' for the 'UK compound' was now fraught with dangers and obstructions: the possibility of unavoidable crowds of people standing in queues or on ferries, borders slamming shut, and the unreliability of our rust bucket Ford Fiesta, which tended to work only when the mood suited it.

So a decision was made, albeit not by me but rather by circumstance. I'd be staying in Sweden. As a storyline arc goes, this was not the most riveting, but with hatches battened, I had no option but to take the Swedish government's fast-developing 'fend for yourself' guidance.

And if there is one thing my life has taught me well, it is how to 'fend'.

My psychotic, self-protecting nature manifested itself in the form of a self-imposed lockdown; a regular top-to-toe coating of alcohol gel and adding a 'o' to any suggested self-distancing measurement. You say, '3 metres', I say, '30'.

Because there were no real guidelines under the auspices of the country I was now trapped in, I did – bearing in mind Sweden's famed self-assembly approach to modern living – build my own lockdown. But just as we had argued over those Netflix flights of fiction, we were now at loggerheads over a documentary in the making. This was, apparently, going to be a lockdown for one.

I deemed the porch area of our flat the 'Contaminated Zone'; it was clearly demarked by the black floor tiles which ended before you entered the corona-free hallway. On a shelf, there was a pump-action bottle of hand gel which I used the moment I entered the flat and before I touched the latch on the cupboard door where I hang my coat. The door to the bathroom was also in the Contaminated Zone, and that could be opened with recently gelled hands before a thorough soap and water scrub up, after which I was free to enter the corona-free hallway. Anything which came through the letterbox could be placed on the shelf next to the hand gel and left for three days where it could decontaminate itself. In an ideal world, I imagined that post-Covid, I'd bury the entire contaminated entrance to our flat in 15 tonnes of concrete, à la Chernobyl.

I felt this secured my immediate surrounds, the unknown factor, however, was the world beyond my front door. We live on the ground floor of a small apartment block, which meant I could use the spy hole in the front door to make sure no potential chatty neighbours were ready to pounce on me in the building's lobby. My body no longer allows me the luxury of dashing, but I soon became adept at swiftly getting to the relative sanctum of the Great Outdoors. The city of Malmö is notoriously windy, a curse which was fast becoming a blessing – no airborne virus had safety in numbers against the endless cyclone which seems to operate around the clock.

I had long since given up going to supermarkets. In addition, I had not used public transport since taking a train and a bus back from the airport after our trip to Thailand.

The only reason I ever really went out was for a daily dose of vitamin D, something I got direct from the source rather than in tablet form from a store (I already take a handful of pills a day, so best not add to that tablet mountain). I took keeping one's distance to an extreme and found myself giving any passer-bys a Titanic-esque wide berth, and if that wasn't possible, I'd hold my breath until a sufficient distance had passed between us.

My Covid Fortress was complete, and my self-protective, psychotic nature dealt with any rogue external factors outside of my control. But I was not as safe as I could've been, my armour still had that chink.

My wife.

Tess had been making tokenistic efforts to work from home but would not shy away from having to pop into the office for, what felt to me like absurdly arbitrary reasons ('I want my cat coffee cup'). She baulked at the cost of online grocery deliveries and wrote off the whole notion of face masks as utterly farcical.

Hers was not an extreme reaction in these parts. During the first few months of the pandemic having arrived in Sweden, if you saw someone wearing a face mask, you'd also see at least two people staring and pointing at them – even the nation's chief epidemiologist (the then 15-minutes'-of-famed Anders Tegnell) was casting serious dispersions on their use.

I would throw an uppity strop every time she clattered through the front door and into the Contaminated Zone laden down by food shopping. To her credit, she did wash her hands before entering the hallway, but only after touching the coat cupboard door with her ungelled Covid-y hands.

I'd lambast her, citing quotes from the most recent fear-mongering scientist who'd just been interviewed on BBC 5 Live. The problem with arguing with Tess over anything remotely science-y, however, is that I enter the debate with a borderline pass in GCSE science, and she enters the debate having studied one semester of chemistry at one of Sweden's most prestigious universities.

That does not make her qualified to govern a nation's pandemic response, but then I probably could not be trusted putting her old lab coat through the correct wash cycle. Not that she works in anything remotely connected to that rogue semester of nerdery, but it is enough to quash my argument that we should start shampooing with ammonia (or whatever the latest quasi-clever clogs on Twitter was suggesting).

*****

A few weeks after I had been politely requested to work from home, I found myself once again streaming a BBC news service as a stony-faced Boris Johnson took to a Downing Street podium. Effectively, whatever he had to say bore no relevance to my life here in Sweden, but despite any of Sweden's supposed logic, I was now fully ensconced in my birth country's line of defence.

In a desperate bid to stimy deaths, Johnson and his cronies had devised a list of who was most at risk of succumbing to the deadlier end of the Covid spectrum. They were to be sent a letter or a text, all 1.5 million of 'em, detailing how they should live their lives for, what seemed to be at the time, the foreseeable future.

I watched the broadcast, attentively and dutifully.

I was gonna make that list, I was sure of it. I've never been so agog to a BBC news portal. And there I was, not just on the list, but right smack at the *very top* of it. Quite a moment. It is rare for me to top a list, but now is my time – and what a time it was. If I was there in the UK, there would have been a bullet with my name on it.

'Number 1 – solid organ transplant recipients'. And with my two transplanted organs, my position at the top of the list was sealed.

If I were in the UK, the advice would be for me to not only stay at home but also avoid going within 'three steps' of my own wife. Meanwhile, in Sweden, I could have been allowed to go to a restaurant, although the nation had been advised that buffets in lunch restaurants should be avoided ... if there was a queue. So instead of being in the UK with a bullet with my name on, I was in Sweden, with a buffet with my name on.

Through various forums I would read about the purgatory my UK-dwelling fellow transplantees were embarking on. The most vulnerable in society were being instructed to stay in for twelve weeks, no strolling around the garden or popping to the nearest pond to feed the ducks. 'In' meant 'in', although permission was granted for them to open a window. Open a window.

They were being sent food parcels once a week; undeniably an admirable act of benevolence on the part of the UK Government, but I spend a lot of time and energy showing the world I am capABLE, and I am not sure how I would have felt being reduced to accept such charity. Some friends told me they received artwork from local children in the food boxes. They didn't specify whether these works were made from edible glitter on edible rice paper, but if not, then what was the point of them?

(One transplant friend was advised by her local health authority to get someone else to take her bins out, that is a piece of guidance I would have been quite happy for Sweden to adopt.)

All of a sudden, it was dawning on me that I had had a lucky escape from the UK-located community in the compound. Here in Sweden, I was able to get fresh air every day when I so desired, and sure, Tess might have been taking our lives into her hands when she went to the local supermarket, but at least she came home with fresh food and *not* a crayoned stick man doing a double thumbs-up with a speech bubble that says 'Thinking of you' scrawled out by a totally random kid. Tess and I actively chose not to have children; I'd say pretending to like crappy artwork was probably low but among the list of reasons we made that choice.

Friends and family in the UK were getting increasingly fearful for my predicament, presumably a fear spurned on by what they could see going on around them as their country descended into, what appeared to be, a dystopic film noir.

Meanwhile, in one UK newspaper headline, the Swedish government was accused of playing Russian roulette with its population. I couldn't seem to avoid gun metaphors where I was not in the firing line with a crosshair on my forehead.

For Tess, the pressure was mounting. Had she not been privy to a constant onslaught of UK fearmongering and soundbites which screamed from my computer screen and speakers that the end was nigh, she might have never changed her course. However, eavesdropping on conversations between my mother and I, Tess would have picked up on the level of concern everyone back in the UK had for me.

I am not quite sure what the tipping point for her was, but on the tenth of April, I was invited to my first ever non-work Zoom group chat. It was with one of my oldest friends and a few of his mates whom I've gotten to know over the years.

It was back when both the pandemic and Zoom were a bit of a novelty – at least two of us thought it was absolutely hysterical to appear in the chat wearing face masks. It was taking us a while to get our heads into this new form of socialising and during one lapse in conversation, a silence-filling question was thrown to the digital floor:

'Does anyone know anyone who has actually had *it*?'

(There was only one '*it*' now, and 'it' was to remain 'it' for quite some time.)

Personally, I only knew of friends of colleagues who had so far succumbed, but it was not long before a name was proffered to the group: some bloke, who one of the Zoomers knew through a local theatre group. It took a while for a few memories to be prodded before three of the five of us cottoned on that they did indeed know him in some vague capacity or another.

Fourteen days after that 'meeting', a local newspaper based in the town where I grew up, shared an article on its Facebook timeline reporting the death of a much-loved man with links to a local theatre group. People were starting to die, and while I did not know this guy, the social circles which divided us were actually more like a Venn diagram.

The man's death, Machiavellian-y or otherwise, was used to further lobby Tess to join me and make this a lockdown for two.

*****

At this point, there was no real evidence as to how transplant patients around the world were faring. Tales of fit young 30-somethings, however, with no underlying health issues who had spluttered and gargled their last words to a remotely located and devastated family down an iPad lent to them by the NHS were making the headlines in the UK. Similar tales were doing the same in Sweden. My battle was won, although it did take rather a high death toll to achieve it: Tess locked herself down.

In reality, there were more restrictions here beyond curbing the 'all you can eat' lunch trade. Social gatherings were, later rather than sooner, limited to fifty people, although schools for the under-16s remained open – a Canadian friend living in Sweden actually received an angry letter from her local authorities after she pulled her kids out of school. But I am not a schoolboy, and I can't remember when I was at a social gathering with more than a handful of people. These new rules didn't match my own self-imposed protectionism.

Sweden's approach was still being internationally regarded as a mad social experiment; from the outside, it looked like the government was turning a blind eye, but the Swedes – and I was now starting to agree – were looking at a world in lockdown, scratching their heads and pondering, 'I'm sorry, *who* is conducting the mad experiment?'.

Sweden was not actually turning a blind eye, far from it, but the difference lied between 'encourage' and 'enforce'. We were 'encouraged' to social distance, work from home and protect the vulnerable. The onus of responsibility lied far more heavily here on the individual. I know I'm vulnerable, so I protected myself.

Throughout the first half of 2020, the only time I truly felt at risk, ironically, was when I had to go to the hospital. As it stood, I needed to go there once a month for a routine blood test. The first time I had to do this after the pandemic kick-off, I was the only one in the entire room who, including both the hospital staff and the pre-blood-letted public, wore a face mask (and we'll get to the full story of *that* mask later). They had introduced a booking system, replacing their normal drop-in policy, to keep numbers down, but it felt like scant protection, bearing in mind everyone in the room was either highly likely to come in contact with the disease (the staff) or die of it (the patients).

The stares I got for wearing that mask said everything about how the Swedes clung to every word their chief epidemiologist said. Anders Tegnell had fast become a household name, not just in Sweden, but also across the world.

He would pop up on various news channels to diplomatically explain why he thought Sweden was taking the most logical approach. The fact that he bore more than a passing resemblance to The Muppet Show's scientist Beaker was adding to his cult appeal. Anders's face was appearing on tote bags and t-shirts; as a 'brand', he was probably about as viral as corona itself. He had decreed the face mask as being more harmful than helpful, and that's all the Swedes needed to hear.

It was the return cycle from that blood test, however, that proved pivotal in my thought process. Spring had sprung and I felt no immediacy to race back to the warmth of our home to keep out of the elongated Swedish winter. I took a detour to maintain my daily exercise routines, and as I did so, I saw buses of people going to work. I had seen photos shared on social media of deserted UK streets, but here in Sweden, life resembled some kind of normality. There was a municipal worker aboard a lawn mower, spraying the scent of freshly-cut grass in his wake; with no face masks to dampen the smell in sight and with no one looking the remotest bit anxious about that fact, it really did serve as quite the mood boost. I had never valued my freedom so much.

*****

We all knew that no one country had a long-term solution to this, but as 2020 rolled on, it became obvious to me that the Swedish flag was the optimal one to be living under. This disease might be left to run slightly more amok through this country, but, as the world seemed to teeter on the precipice of a global depression, was it so wrong to have one eye on the health of the nation and the other on the economy?

Was it so naïve of them to consider the implications and inevitable death toll of a workforce in lockdown alongside deaths caused directly by The Virus itself?

When the UK Clap for Carers initiative began and the UK stood in solidarity on their doorsteps to applaud the collective efforts of the front-liners, were they picturing those doctors and nurses with/without PPE, beads of sweat forming on their visor-protected brows, or one year, two, five, twenty years in the future, battling a tsunami of mental health issues, an onslaught of alcohol-induced organ failures, an obesity crisis, unprecedented levels of drug addiction and tending to those left bereft by suicide?

Or maybe I was wrong, and Sweden was on the cusp of a historic massacre. Time had yet to tell. Meanwhile, I was happy to head out on my bike every day with the sun on my face, just because I could.

*****

The more we plunged into this pandemic, the more epoch defining it began to feel. I was even starting to sense it may further divvy up our long-standing Gregorian calendar. Will western history books now talk about Before Christ, Anno Domini, Normal and New Normal? I guess that depends on whether we were to have a future from which we could reflect upon this history-in-the-making catastrophuck.

Either way, everything was seemingly in a constant flux of topsy-turvying. What was once routine was now out of the question, and what was never questioned was now forbidden from our routine.

I started to notice how the humble greeting 'you al-right?' was beginning to carry more gravitas. No matter what prompted the question, the answer used to be practically the knee-jerk same: 'Yeah, fine thanks'.

But who could lay claim to being 'fine thanks' during a pandemic? Every 'fine thanks' needed further contextualising, '... yer know, considering'. In light of my newfound at-easeness, friends had started to wonder, bearing in mind my personal circumstances, 'What the hell does he have to be so happy about?'.

On the face of it, the fact that my health conditions render me a sitting duck with a broken wing, limp-waddling through a shooting range should be enough to temper my mood. On top of that, I had not only inflicted a bespoke self-isolation upon myself but also been forcefully segregated from my UK-residing family and friends – to whom I am a regular visitor. Those trips are pivotal to my mental well-being.

In theory, I had the worst of so many worlds.

So, what gives?

Truth is, when it comes to isolating, I am a past master. I've felt depths of isolation I doubt the pandemic could ever have plummeted to. Not even close. While it was the very same UK-based family and friends who provided me with so much support during my years of ill-health, the reality is that loitering around the porch of death's door is truly a lonely experience.

Death's door is, from my vantage point, one way: it only lets one in at a time, has no exit, offers no group discount, has no fire escape (even in the flame-y bit) and is surprisingly disabled-friendly.

So, while I might have been surrounded by the best of company, I knew no one was going to cross that threshold with me. The ultimate petrifying isolation.

That door doesn't go away once you know its GPS location, but post-transplant, I've retreated down the crazy-paved pathway which leads to it. How I ended up married, and living and working in Sweden after all that still baffles me, but here I am. But those baffling circumstances led to a whole new breed of isolation.

I am 'an English bloke' in 'a Swedish office'. I have formed some wonderful friendships there, but these friendships thrive in small groups or one-to-one dynamics. Good for me. My Swedish language skills can ably navigate me through many an everyday secondary school-standard oral test situation, but the machinations of a bureaucratic meeting, or the nuances of coffee-break bantz? I am often left lost for (Swedish) words. Isolated by my own laziness and ignorance, well, yes, but isolated all the same. Surrounded by friends and friendly faces, but as isolated as ever.

But now it seemed I'd been 'saved by the hell' – lockdowns and self-isolations were my liberation. My own time-management had been handed to me on a sterilised, sterling silver platter, and I was happy to lick it cleaner.

While the option was there to take our work breaks and drink coffee over Zoom, I instead found myself 'zoom'-ing down the coastal cycle paths of southern Sweden, choosing not to take my screen breaks sat in front of a screen, which I am fairly sure is the point of them.

The cutting blade of the Swedish winter was soon totally dulled by the Swedish spring. Where once I was sat awkwardly on the lunch sofa, mentally exhausting myself as I tried to keep up with whatever Netflix series I must binge/ avoid (often I wasn't sure due to my piss-poor Swedish), I now found myself conversing only with my inner dialogue. And boy, do we agree on what to watch next.

What have I got to be so happy about? I'd ponder to myself, with the sun on my SPF 50-protected face, blossoming lilac bushes one side of me and the ebbing sea on the other. At that moment, I couldn't possibly imagine!

I know my isolations, and believe me, the pandemic-induced one was the best so far.

FOR THE (MEDICAL) RECORD

In the early stages of my ill-health, I hardly cut the typical figure of an international man of mystery, certainly not as I hobbled down eastern European cobbled streets on my NHS crutches wearing a grubby, and at times bloodied eye patch, or when I was sat in a wheelchair and hydraulically lifted to the entrance of a waiting budget airline jet, but despite my stricken circumstances, there was no doubt about it – I got around ... albeit slowly and unsurely.

As injury and illness finally got the better of me, such buccaneering was put on hold, but wowzers, what a much-needed wake-up call it all was! Even as a shrinking violet of a traveller, I could not avoid the tirade of justified social, historical and political accusations levelled at me, based purely on my nationality.

I never really questioned what was wrong with being both British and simultaneously abroad, but the world decided to explain it to me anyway. I was once offered to participate in a fist fight by a Belgian simply because he overheard me ordering a white wine in English ('yer knowz, footballz and thingz, you like the fight, non?'). A disgruntled Croatian girlfriend, in a fit of disappointment, once proclaimed the scowling put-down 'ne pravi se Englez'. Turns out that in the Balkans, if you do something entirely illogical, baffling and against any sense of reason, you are accused of 'acting like the English'.

As we waded into the deeper waters of the pandemic, I was missing England more than ever, at least the pre-Covid version of it. The fact that my two passport-issuing nations were at odds about what I should be doing with myself was starting to bother me and land me in some awkward conversations, particularly as one of the nation's was being a bit judge-y about the other.

In reality, as spring became summer, I was often to be found lazing around in one of the city's parks or on the beach. On one particular afternoon, I was out sitting in the shadow of a windmill with 20-plus colleagues eating picnic food and boozily toasting the beckoning Midsummer Day, after which many Swedes disappear from work for about a month. Later in the week, a similar event was held on the beach to watch the sunset, all made safe by a bring-your-own blanket/glass/mug/fuck-off-you-are-too-close-to-me glare policy, and, of course, lashings and lashings of alcohol gel.

This was in the same week that Sweden made UK headlines after the World Health Organization listed it among eleven countries which were, and I'll paraphrase, 'pandemically fucked'. Sweden normally hovers around lists which boast advanced welfare systems or the best places to live, but now it seemingly sat among countries run by crazed despots or with seriously dodgy human rights records.

As I was becoming accustomed to, I received a trickle of concerned correspondence from my UK friends and family. One could only assume that they were unaware that just days after the WHO made that statement, they checked their facts, backtracked and took Sweden off the list – 'Sweden is actually doing okay', is, after all, a shit headline.

Sweden is geographically vast, but by population, rather puny. Statistics were being broken down by region, and one week, in the southern tip where I live, one of the days recorded -3 deaths. -3. This was due to an uncharacteristic bureaucratic error rather than a mutation of the virus which had now taken us into the 'reanimation zombie phase'.

So, I guess I felt safe enough here, where I was free to roam, and I guess I'd feel safe if I'd been in government-enforced solitary confinement in the UK. What irked me a little was quite how quick the UK media were to point at and criticise other nations. A little colonial superiority complex hangover, perhaps, or just another justification for 'ne pravi se Englez'?

Chapter 6
You snuffle, I snuff it

A-a-a-tishoo

Really?

Aaaaaatishoo

You have got to be taking the piss?

'tishoo

Well, that's put my next few weeks in jeopardy.

My. Heart. Sinks.

Can you even imagine? A dinner party participant leans back on their chair, laces their fingers behind their head, makes a nonchalant but ultimately futile effort to tilt their face away, and jettisons three snot scuds across the table.

No biggie for any of the other invitees, gauging from the complete lack of reaction. This was in December 2019, when such table manners, while most certainly should have at the very least been considered 'fucking appalling', were not given the life-threatening status they would be granted just three or four months later.

But it was a biggie for me, and – globally – millions like me. I live in fear of The Sneeze and have done so ever since my body became overly reliant on immune-suppressant medications. A cold for you is like the flu for me, and the flu for you is, for me, like ... well, you just have to visit your local intensive care ward to see how this particular analogy ends.

Those three sneezes took place around the time a Wuhan woman working in that now infamous 'wet market' got back home from a long day of dolloping out ladles of sea horse foetus soup and announced to her husband, 'I've got that tickle in the back of my throat, yer know, the one I get when I am coming down with something'. Or, as the best guessers were soon to name her, Patient Zero.

It was the run up to Christmas – a time when it becomes increasingly difficult to avoid alpha males who've 'braved it' to the office party despite sounding like their nose needs to be industrially-dredged or children germ carpet-bombing their vicinities while off their collective noggins on cheap, powdery, Santa-shaped chocolate.

I've been living on high alert for years, and now so are you. Rubbish, isn't it? Me and the millions were joined by healthy, bouncy billions, and it looked like we were all in this pandemic purgatory together and, as we ride the waves as they ebb and flow, the long haul.

The Millions are made up of quite the spectrum of conditions, everyone from perky, pony-tailed Insta-influencers who detail their pregnancies granola bowl by granola bowl, to 'mummy, mummy why doesn't that woman have any hair?' stage four liver cancer patients.

Despite our multitude, The Millions are relatively quiet. The Billions couldn't wait to yank their super-spreader kids out of school the minute there was a whiff of corona in a hundred-mile radius of the catchment area. But ever stop to think about the pre-corona age mum on her fifth round of chemo who had to send her three kids to primary school in full knowledge that your kid could sneeze on her kid, that kid could get a cold and pass it on to mum, who could subsequently develop chronic pneumonia and ...

Die.

That isolation you've now felt, the frustration that you couldn't or can't do exactly what you please whenever you choose; that fear, that fear that, despite all the odds and all the evidence-based research which seemingly screamed 'don't be so ridiculous', you will in fact be knocked from your pedestal of privilege and, well ... like the mum of three, die.

That blip of isolation to you is a lifetime for us. And many of The Millions have a shorter 'use by date' than most of The Billions. You've got time to spare, we ain't.

The Millions carry on regardless and without voice. The Billions have the power to grind the global economy to a pitiful halt, a shift which will inevitably shunt a proportion of The Millions, a greater proportion of which live either in, or on the brink of, poverty to an even earlier grave.

I guess that is, in some global-evolutionary perspective, fair enough. Like Darwinism's Ferrari crashing into Democracy's Volkswagen – both agree it's just collateral damage on humanity's journey. So, while the actions of The Billions will lead to the deaths of many of The Millions, we'll just have to live with it. Besides, speaking as one of The Millions, I am actually rather happy you've finally joined us.

That is not a sentiment borne out of spite, more one of relief, really. The safer you keep yourselves, the safer you keep us. I said nothing when those sneeze droplets, possibly neutralised by their alcohol-intoxicated nasal cannon, settled where the dessert was soon to be served. Can you imagine the members of The Billions who sat around that table saying nothing if that were to happen now? Not likely.

*****

I sometimes think I am the walking, talking, haemorrhaging version of the boardgame Operation. I've been sliced and spliced and lasered and lanced so many times I'm not even sure what qualifies as a bona fide operation and what is just a medical procedure. I don't, for example, count the insertion of my dialysis line into my gut as proper surgery despite that I still sport a scar from the scalpel. Maybe I've just become too hardened, but if it can be done under a local anaesthetic, then it just doesn't count, at least it doesn't in my ledger book.

I tend to refer to the transplant surgery, as and when is necessary or appropriate (and I do my utmost to reduce the number of 'as and whens'), as 'the big operation' – just a conversational tool for those who know me that I am not referring to one of my other myriad surgeries.

I was an inpatient for 14 days before I was hoofed out by means of a wheelchair ride through the hospital's revolving doors to start my convalescence – hardly a break for freedom, and it wouldn't be long before those doors were rotating me back in.

Leaving the transplant ward is akin to ending a relationship with a particularly needy and clingy partner after what you thought, or at least hoped, had been a clean and amicable parting. They still wanted to see me. All. The. Bloody. Time. 'Aww, c'mon Adrian. Come back. I want to see you again, I have some stuff I want to talk about. I just want to make sure you're okay, go through a few things with you, yer know?' Not quite how the appointment letters from my consultant were worded, but that is how they were read.

(Of course, that analogy could be flipped on its head; maybe I was just kicked out for being too independent. Maybe they saw the fact that I could now walk without a zimmer frame, wash my own face and genitals, wipe my own bum, use my mouth as an entry point to consume food rather than a tube into my chest as a slight to their hospitality. Maybe they were tired of me telling them that I could do things without them nagging. Although it doesn't take long before you miss being handed sweet cups of tea on the hour or, at your beck and call, someone to plump up your pillow, fresh sheets every day, every whim of your neediness being met with a warm, friendly smile, and, of course, my hospital crush, Pharmacy Girl.)

Left to my own devices (which now no longer included a dialysis machine), I am, quite frankly, an excellent patient. I have an alarm set on my phone to notify me of when to gobble down my pills, and I am borderline neurotic about taking them. I hang on the every word of nurses, doctors, consultants, specialists, anyone wearing scrubs, really, and attend every follow-up appointment with the due diligence of a try-hard teacher's pet.

It all stemmed from my newfound fear of rejection. Despite me brimming with optimism and energy, I was ever conscious of the very real possibility of my body reacting to the new organs as some kind of alien invasion. That fear still haunts me, it lurks behind every thought I have; it lurks in my subconscious mind like the shadow of a great white shark beneath my inflatable Lilo. Ever present.

I'd be back as an outpatient three times a week for the first few months post-big op and would find myself sitting in a waiting room surrounded by people who were all on the same journey as me. I've learned to curate carefully who I talk to about my condition, particularly when it comes to those in the same precarious situation. I didn't want my zeal quashed by a sob story from a recent transplant recipient who was now weeks away from their body booting out their pilfered organs.

There is a spectrum of people I tend to avoid, a spectrum which includes those who consider transplant surgery as a 'miracle' and not the painstaking and pioneering work of scientists and surgeons. I am not sure what kind of miracle-performing god would choose to save my life while throwing another man from his motorbike and leaving him just a crimson stain of jumbled limbs and piss and shit-soiled leathers on a motorway for a team of surgeons to later harvest for 'anything worth keeping'.

At the other end of the spectrum are – and this is painful to admit – the ones who came out of this surgery far more visibly scarred than I did.

In those waiting rooms, I kept myself to myself, conversing only with my mother's partner, Barry, who had seemingly taken on the responsibility of ferrying me to my steady stream of appointments and blood tests. But sometimes the conversation comes to you, and there is one particular conversation which burned into my psyche.

We were sitting adjacent to an elderly lady who was happily, and rather audibly, engaged in chat with an apparent stranger. She was elegantly dressed, well-spoken and clearly adept at delivering her anecdote. It didn't sound like the first time she had regaled it.

'I've had as many transplants as I've had husbands', she quipped. She had, from all accounts, now had the second kidney for quite some time, and it was working 'ticketyboo'. I noticed she now had the ear of most of this particular corner of the waiting room. She continued, 'I rejected my first kidney and my first husband at the same time'. Only a practiced orator can make such a line sound amusing, but it was told with a wry smile and the 'audience' reacted accordingly.

But it was the conclusion of her anecdote which still haunts me to this very day. Her first husband, who she was seemingly never quite sure about in the first place, had taken her to the cinema to see a film she didn't care to watch. She went on to tell of a man, sitting close to where her and her then husband sat, sneezing the whole way through the film. Within weeks she had succumbed to a flu which had then triggered her body into rejecting her first kidney.

Have you ever sneezed in a cinema? I know I have, who hasn't?

Of course I cannot verify the medical validity or the biological machinations of her claim, but it didn't, and still doesn't, matter. When people around the same dinner table as me sneeze, it is that woman and her tale of woe that I think of. She didn't die, clearly, but the idea of me rejecting my beloved new organs due to someone sneezing at me, or even near me, fills me with, quite frankly, a very red and misty rage.

In my mind, we are all on countdown clocks to our own demise, and I am fairly sure when I was living for all those years with a broken pancreas and banjaxed kidneys, that countdown clock was counting down in double-quick time. My lifestyle now is very much geared around slowing that countdown clock down. I could do without any friend or foe, or colleague or carer inadvertently tinkering with my clock cogs.

*****

I get the impression that the fact that I can pick up a virus with the apparent ease of my mother's laptop labels me as 'the sickly type'. But the truth is, in the seven years I have been back in the world of work, I've only had a handful of days off as a result of succumbing to a rogue virus.

While I am part of the immune-compromised masses, that compromise is not a symptom of me being ill, pasty, weak and fragile looking. The truth is that it is self-inflicted, namely the immunosuppressive agents I take to stop my immune system working as well as it might. Left to its own devices, my body would fight off fevers and flus with the best of them, it would also kick out my appropriated organs along the way. That's the 'compromise' I have to live with.

This taints the way I look at the world and The Ables who thrive in it. A colleague, upon hearing I had at one point not worked for seven years straight, boasted that he had never taken a day off sick in his life. Not more than a year later, he fell afoul of cancer and died. As a 40-something living in an image-obsessed world, I am not short

of peers who seem boastfully proud of their youthful –
whether by means of genes, makeup, or filters – fresh and
firm looks. All I can think of is their internal organs. They
can do their best to live as healthier a life as possible, but
all our organs are aging. Inside all of us there is one of our
potential fates yet to unfold. The Ables' countdowns might
not be ticking as fast as mine, but they sure are ticking, and
one thing is for sure, two of my organs are seventeen years
younger than the rest of me; I'd like to think that gives me
an advantage, but it really doesn't.

*****

Despite the fact that in the early 2000s I was granted permission to live in my nan's house after her death, upon
arrival, I was not the only resident. My moving-in date
had been postponed by an eye operation and subsequent
convalescence at my mother's. During this time, the spare
room had been occupied by a friend who needed a place to
stay, conveniently at the same time that my mother needed help to cover the cost of the property.

Mark, the tenant in question, bore witness to the very
early stages of the business end of my illness which had
manifested itself in the form of perpetual vomiting and
mind-crushing migraines. We both spent far too long in
the bathroom, him for preening, me for puking. Despite
the fact that the sicker I became, and the more I felt com-
forted by an on-hand potential ambulance-calling friend, I
was forced by circumstance to ask Mark to leave.

His room, which could squeeze in a double bed, a ward-
robe, and a bedside table, was cleared solely for the storage of my dialysis supplies – chiefly made up of cardboard

boxes piled precariously high which lined three of the walls. The boxes containing the bags of ever-so-slightly gloopy fluid which was pumped into and drained out of me in cycles every night. Each box contained two bags, each bag contained six litres of fluid, and I needed three bags per night.

(Turning an entire room of your house into, what appeared to me, a pharmaceutical storage facility, is a surreally depressing moment, and not one offset by the fact that the local council gave me a discount off my council tax as the room could no longer qualify as a bedroom).

Every day for over a year I had to fetch one box and one extra bag of fluid from the spare room and take it to my bedroom, where the dialysis machine was placed on a table next to my bed. I'd have to set the machine up during the day, when I had the energy to lift the boxes. Once connected, the bags, along with my cat, Milo the Bastard – in flagrant breach of hygiene protocol – would rest on a concave, heated bed on the top of the machine, where they would warm to body temperature.

There was a step down from my bedroom, and across from the top of the stairs there was a step up to the spare room. Not a great distance, even for an ever-weakening soul such as myself.

But those boxes broke me.

What is it you picture when you think of someone with an illness, a disease, or a disability? Epileptics have fits, right? Parkinson's Disease sufferers shake; dementia patients forget stuff; anorexics are skinny, and people who use wheelchairs ... are in wheelchairs.

But what is it you don't think of? Every disease and disability comes with a plague of physical, mental, sociological, logistical, and practical complications. Scale it down to taking a day off work with a cold; in the short term, that might mean letting down a colleague, kids being late for school, dragging yourself to the chemist to buy some Night Nurse. Take a week off work with a bad cold, and you will feel the financial pinch at the end of the month with a docked pay slip; maybe the next month you'll be shopping at Lidl rather than Waitrose to ensure you don't have to dip into the holiday fund. Now scale that up to not working for, in my case, years. But for many others, it's decades, and for some, it's the rest of their lives.

The consequences are unfathomable unless you've had to face them.

Despite failing vision, failing organs, failing finances and a failing relationship, it was those bastard cardboard boxes which ultimately got the better of me.

I had never considered the disposal of cardboard as being such a crippling knock-on effect of double organ failure, but 'crippling' was ultimately what it was, almost. All of a sudden, I had more cardboard than an Amazon packaging plant. I couldn't just throw it away, as that was a fineable offence by my, not green but greenish local authority. I had a large wheelie bin exclusively for such detritus, but two days' worth of discarded dialysis fluid boxes would overwhelm it.

I called my local council and explained the situation, and they eventually supplied me with extra wheelie bins. It must've looked like I was starting my own cottage industry recycling plant to my neighbours, a notion not helped by the fact that the council also provided me with a fluorescent yellow hazardous waste bin.

But the administrative process of disposing of the boxes was not the real issue. My skinny and ever-weakening body had to first flatten them. I am not a practical person, but I can flatten a box, or at least I thought I could. The boxes were made of incredibly tough and reinforced cardboard, and they were further strengthened by – what felt like – industrial-strength glue and gigantic metal staples which looked big and strong enough to repair a bridge.

One morning, as I tried to wrestle a box into a flattened submission, instead of the *box* crumpling, I did. I just couldn't do it. I collapsed onto the box in tears. Perhaps I was not young and hip enough to be on peritoneal dialysis after all. It had not even been a month, but I just couldn't go on like this. My frazzled thoughts weighed up the options. Well, option.

Haemodialysis.

Haemo is what most people think of when they think of people on dialysis. The kind of machine you've probably fundraised for at a Blue Peter bring 'n' buy sale. It's a procedure where the patient is connected to the machine via a permanently inserted and intrusive tube into the arm or neck, and their blood is, effectively, given a spin cycle.

Normal protocol means you have to do this every other day in a hospital or a special dialysis unit. So, reduced independence, a colossal use of your time (not that I needed 'time' anyway), and hours upon hours of being attached to a machine surrounded by my least favourite types of people – people like me. Still, no f-ing boxes, and at that time, that's all I cared about.

(I am not sure if the Ministry of Sick Jokes was closed down as part of Prime Minister David Cameron's 2010 austerity measures, but I do have to confess chortling as a teenager – probably at an age when I was offering up my then-too-small Pepe snow wash jeans for a Blue Peter jumble sale – to the following joke:

Q: What sits at the end of your bed and takes the piss?

A: A kidney dialysis machine.

In fear of being *that* person, the joke just doesn't work. Dialysis machines do not 'take the piss', they clean the blood of toxins that piss contains. If your kidneys fail, you don't piss at all – I did not pass 'clean' or 'dirty' piss for years.

If you want a better joke:

 Q: What did the terrorist do when his kidneys failed?

A: Dial-ISIS' (this does work better but is time sensitive).

Either way, I calmed my emotions and called my mother, who was now my apparent co-pilot on this journey of despair. Understanding my distress, she agreed that, hospital willing, it was my decision. But there was certainly some hesitancy in her voice. Perhaps she just knew that it was not for the best, that the doctors were right to say what form of treatment I should be receiving, but perhaps she also knew that while I was entrusting her with the role of co-pilot, that position actually meant 'chauffeur' in practical terms. She knew by now that hospital transport was scant, and she'd end up sacrificing just as much of her time and as I did mine. At that point, she was working full time, and a significant proportion of her salary was already subsidising some of the gaps in benefit support the UK government overlooked. She could not forego more work hours just to watch her son's blood being painstakingly percolated three times a week.

So boxes it was. And while they had successfully broken my mental resolve, they had not finished with me yet.

By 2008 my feet had been out of casts and medieval torture-esque looking orthotics for over a year, but I was left permanently tentative on my toes. My balance is poor, and every step I took (and am still taking) is laced with caution. But I knew that house inside out. I'd manoeuvre myself around it with all the finesse I could muster, even if that was the finesse one would expect of a daddy long legs with elephantiasis in two of its legs.

Despite that, on one fateful morning not long after I had finally mastered the art of box crumpling (using my entire body as a dead weight was the key), I was scraping my energy resource's barrel to prep my dialysis machine. While carrying a box and a bag of dialysis fluid, I misstepped from one bedroom to another. I crunched down on my heel for what would have been a 'whoopsie' moment for most but was a cold rush of blood to the head and to the heel for me.

Days later, I was back in a cast, in which I would remain for the greater share of the year and five months I was on dialysis. I had cleanly broken the heel bone of my right foot. The emergency cord on 'wheelchair use' was pulled. One day, my mother arrived to take me on a supermarket excursion in a rather nifty looking wheelchair. Turns out that a husband of a friend of a friend of my mum had bought the lightweight bit of kit and never got around to using it before dying of motor neurone disease – that's certainly one up from the 'one careful lady owner' you might come across when shopping for a set of new wheels. The purchase was secured by a donation to the most relevant (and requested) charity.

So it was the boxes which pushed me over the edge, both physically and mentally. As a whodunnit mystery, surely 'the cardboard boxes in the bedroom' would be low down the list of suspects.

On May 15th, 2009, and by the time that the anaesthetist prepped me for 'the big operation', my body, mental health, spirit, and soul had been smashed to smithereens. The usual guff about the low odds of dying while under the knife had been dictated to me, as it had been so many times prior. So while my thoughts upon waking were more of a soiled-sheets scatological nature, the thoughts I had moments before I went under were more profound and philosophical: I had become totally at ease with this being the end, this being the final time I felt and smelt that now oh-so-familiar gust of anaesthetic blasting into my face – if I were never to wake and die mid drug-induced blissful slumber, then so be it. I was cool with that.

*****

So what do you think about when you know you are just about to come down with anything on the lurgy spectrum? Might not be able to join your mates for that pint tomorrow night (maybe you will go either way), might miss that work meeting (you'll probably go, but straight home and to bed after), might miss choir rehearsal (you're the lead tenor, you can hardly bail on it). All *I* think about is doom, disability, dialysis and, while I do my best to prevent it shadowing my every thought, death.

We're all finally and depressingly on the same side, and if I can once again speak on behalf of The Millions, we won't sneeze on you if you don't sneeze on us. Deal?

Chapter 7
How physical fitness destroyed
my mental health

A paradoxical quirk of being on a transplant waiting list is quite how healthy one must be, while at the same time also being in the possession of a kaput vital organ, or, in my case, two kaput vital organs (or, depending on how you count them, three – my two kidneys and one pancreas being busted).

To prove you have the correct equilibrium of being both at death's door but also capable of knocking on that door then running away before Death himself answers, one must undergo a series of physical tests. That might sound like a Channel 4 Bear Grylls kind of challenge, but I'd happily zipline naked into Arctic waters splashing down to a waiting pod of malnourished killer whales than go through that ordeal again.

So, first and foremost, to even be considered for one of the most exclusive VIP (Very Ill People) waiting lists, you must first prove you're, well, a failure. Examinations have never been one of my strongest suits, so failing was something I was used to: both kidneys failed – tick; pancreas failed – tick. So far, so ... good?!

I had already started dialysis when the next set of physical tests commenced. From a psychological perspective, being on a transplant waiting list is a curious void. Unlike, perhaps, the post-death afterlife limbo we have been introduced to via various horror franchises, the Waiting List is the pre-death version of the same limbo, but with one fundamental difference – a very real chance to get back into the fully functioning World of the Living.

Ideally, no one should be on that list, but the very fact that the whole concept contains the word 'waiting' does glean you with some hope. It gives it a sense of a mere temporary status, and while that might be one of the most tortuous moments of anyone's life who has had the misfortune to be on that list, one must cling to the hope that that's all it actually is – a 'moment'.

I cannot recall what expectations I had of how long I would be on that list, but it never really occurred to me that once I was on it, I could be kicked off it; that access would, at one point, be denied. Whether that was just wilful ignorance or my unconscious mind doing its best to protect itself, I guess I'll never know.

As became apparent, however, I might have overdone it with the 'failing'.

*****

I am not sure of my general level of fitness before I became ill. I have always had the physical appearance of a mop – a look I have both embraced and been resigned to as the decades have passed. Tallish and skinny, some years I would swim every week, sometimes I'd not do any physical exercise for months on end. I can't remember what stage I was at when my kidneys started to falter.

One of the tests I needed to undertake was on my heart. They needed to know that it was strong enough to undergo more than ten hours of surgery (just lying there unconscious on an operating table, as it transpires, requires a lot more from your body than you might give it credit for, as does lazing around in bed as you recuperate). I was actually quite looking forward to this test, as I was told I was required to eat a fatty meal just beforehand. I had been on a steadily increasingly insanely restrictive diet for years at this point, and the possibility I could gorge guilt-free on a Marks and Sparks BLT or a Burger King Chicken Royale was positively an oasis of joy in the gastronomical barren desert I had been wandering through.

FOR THE (MEDICAL) RECORD

If having to be fit and fiddly enough – while at the same time needing a dialysis machine and a daily bucket of drugs to stay alive – to be on a waiting list seems counter-intuitive, then the diet you have to maintain while 'waiting' seemingly takes on a whole new level of what-the-fuckery.

Beyond the fads, there are some rudimentary basics to a balanced diet one might employ to maintain a healthy body. But when your body is not healthy, the diet is certainly not balanced.

For example, keeping hydrated is always a good idea, right? The NHS certainly thinks so:

'Water is a healthy and cheap choice for quenching your thirst at any time. It has no calories and contains no sugars that can damage teeth'.

You can't go wrong with water, unless of course the water goes in, but your body has no biological means of getting it back out again.

In the early days of my kidney failure, a doctor asked me, what seemed at the time, a bit of a peculiar question: 'Do your socks leave a mark on your leg when you take them off?' The answer was yes, but I just thought my socks were too tight or had shrunk in the wash. In reality, the puff in my ankles was actually, well, piss – at least it should have been piss (although the doctors call it 'oedema'), my piss overshot the normal exit route, and I was quite literally filling up, feet first.

Before I knew it, the water levels were rising, and my skinny chicken legs filled out to the proportion of a Tour de France cyclist. For the first time ever in my life, my Levi´s 501s actually looked pretty good on me.

For a point of reference, a litre of water weighs one kilo, which is the weight of a bag of sugar, and I was wading around in my own skin with about five litres in each leg. It was then that my blood pressure crashed the hospital's measuring device, doctors feared for my day-to-day chances of survival, and when I collapsed in a heap on a hospital corridor floor, the most obvious conclusion to jump to was that I was having a heart attack.

Once drained by dialysis, I was ordered to consume no more than one and half litres of water a day. And you have no idea how little that is until you've tried to hydrate yourself on that dribble. Common practice is to suck on ice cubes, sometimes I made them a 'treat' by adding sugar-free cordial. The Joy.

I'd nodded my way through my first visit to the hospital's dietician. She at no point questioned my attention. I was permanently thinking through the pea-soup fog my brain was now currently and permanently lost in, but perhaps my speccy look mislead her into thinking I knew what the hell potassium and phosphorous were – she never questioned whether I was taking it all in.

If I'd been asked to add them to my food, I'd have probably gone to the chemist and expected to be handed two test tubes of bubbling, steaming fluid. But I was being asked to take them out of my diet, so I guess in some shape or form, I was already ingesting them.

As it turns out, they're pretty hard to avoid, particularly if you want to eat a conventional, balanced diet. Gone were bananas, oranges, spinach, broccoli, potatoes, mushrooms, peas, baked beans, kidney beans, soybeans, cucumbers, courgette – just a selection from a pretty conventional shopping list, and that's just the stuff with potassium in.

To reduce phosphorous, you've also gotta cut out wholemeal bread, dairy, chicken, turkey, nuts, and a whole bunch of other stuff which I don't eat anyway, like seafood and pork.

Of course, that leaves the snack aisle wide open to abuse, unless of course your pancreas, as mine was, is poleaxed. Mars bars were reserved for medical emergencies only: 'a Mars a day helps you work, rest and ...' avoid a diabetic coma.

My entire dialysis diet was bland, over-cooked and washed down with a thimbleful of water. The mouth-watering prospect that I could soon be chomping down on *that* Marks and Sparks BLT or a Burger King Chicken Royale was, quite literally, just what the doctor ordered.

*****

But burger or bacon sandwich denied. Unfortunately, as my mother was in firm control of when I shopped (and indeed what aisle she decided to roll me down – my local supermarket's wheelchairs were controlled by the walkers, not the rollers), any notion of a one-off binge was off the menu. She had driven me to the appointment and presented me with a homemade cheese sandwich – that was to be my 'fatty meal'. It didn't even have any mayo in it. The fact that I can still recall that detail, I hope demonstrates the deep dissatisfaction I felt.

A deep dissatisfaction, which absolutely paled into a snowstorm of despair, as days later I was told my heart was not strong enough to undergo transplant surgery. Both the words 'waiting' and 'list' were copied and cut from my medical status – my status had gone from 'temporary' to 'terminal'.

I cannot remember how that made me feel, my brain has decided to wipe that from its memory banks; possibly carefully curated selected amnesia, more realistically, I was so used to bad news back then that 'you'll spend the rest of your – now comparatively short – life on dialysis' probably just blended in with the rest of the blow after blow I'd had to absorb into my increasingly frail body and mind.

Forgetting that feeling, along with the look on my mother's face, who had presumably once again driven me to the appointment to hear that news, is a blessing, although if these memories are collated somewhere in my subconscious mind, then I hope my brain has also sectioned it off with razor wire, foaming at the mouthguard dogs and machine gun posts – I never want to accidentally stumble across those memories. Ever.

As a last-ditch attempt to save my life, my heart was subjected to a more thorough investigation, this time by the means of an angiogram. While that involved the insertion of a tube into the main artery in my leg and shoving it up until it reached my heart, what I recall the most – despite how horrific that procedure sounded to my ears – was having my pubes hacked off with a seemingly blunt Bic razor which was being rinsed under cold water. That, and the palpable sense of relief on my mother's face as it contorted back from its more recent incarnation of 'fraught fear' to the stressed, but not stroke-inducing 'perma-panic' that had been her 'look' for more than a year now. I was told that the first test was wrong. My heart was fine, and I could be placed straight back on the waiting list – move directly past 'Go' but consider that your last 'Chance' card.

It was a near miss that has forever haunted me. I know how quickly one minor health glitch can snowball and then avalanche into a life-threatening disaster. I know that either today, tomorrow, next year, or in ten or thirty years' time, there is every chance I will be back under the knife. But this time, I'll be ready for that knife, or at least physically braced for it. I felt that if I was to survive this, I'd get fit and stay fit as soon as I could.

Post-transplant, and ever since starting to feel abso-bloody-lutely amazing, I have maintained a borderline obsessive eye on my health, albeit in a rather stealth manner (I have never been to a gym, I don't own a pair of trainers, or any sportswear at all, now I come to think about it), and that manner has been more than nurtured by apparent health-fixated/outdoors-y Swedish lifestyle norms.

*****

Driving is now a dim and distant memory. When I return to the UK, I am entirely dependent on public transport, taxis and cadged lifts from family and friends. There is something rather humbling and humiliating about always having to rely on others as a mode of transport. Of course anyone ferrying me around is doing me a huge favour, but questions such as 'Shall I drop you here?' and 'When's a good time to pick you up?' leave me feeling rather infantilised.

But in Sweden, everything is flipped on its head. I live in one of the most cycle-friendly cities in the world. And cycling is not only one of the few things my body can do, but also it's something my podiatrist actively encourages me to do — the less time I spend on my feet, the better, and anything which is non-weight bearing is good to go as far as she is concerned.

Not only that, but far from being the pain-in-the-backside-friend/son/brother who always needs collecting from the station – as I am in the UK – thanks to the fact that I decided to buy myself a shiny, new, black bike (deemed by the local scumbags as the most desirable to nick), I am now the pushbike equivalent of 'that wanker in a Ferrari'. The bicycle was a present for myself, from myself, which I bought in 2015 after receiving my first proper wage packet post-transplant.

Now, every journey I make starts with me unlocking my bike. It is how I get to and from work, it is how I get to and from my social life, and it is how I get to and (struggle) back from the supermarket laden down with a weekly shop precariously balanced on the rack over my back wheel. It is also part of my keep-me-out-from-under-the-knife healthy lifestyle choices. Sure, the exercise does me good, but during the winter (and while my colleagues put this down to the behaviour of an eccentric 'Brit' who cycles to work through a snowstorm), it keeps me away from the virus-laden plumes of breath which hang heavy in the buses.

In fact, I actually have two bicycles now. The shiny black one named Shep, due to the fact that it is made by the Swedish company Skeppshult (a brand which if mispronounced badly enough, lends itself to sounding like 'Sheps-hult'), and of course a nod to the loyalty of the BBC children's telly presenter John Noakes's faithful canine companion, who was also called Shep.

I also have Herman, called so because the now long-gone Swedish brand which originally manufactured it named the model 'Hermes'. Herman is over 85 years old, has no gears, barely discernible brakes, steers like an oil tanker, is used only in the summer months, and is perhaps one of my most loved inanimate objects. It was a birthday gift from the Swedish Wife.

As it turns out, when I am not in the UK being infantilised as a perpetual passenger, I infantilise myself by naming my bicycles.

*****

In 2020, it was only when I first ventured out to my first hospital appointment post-self-imposed lockdown that I realised quite how much I missed the combination of both fresh air and cycling. Prior to that, I had been carpet-bombing my psyche with doom-laden news, as ever from the UK, which often featured images of empty streets and shuttered shops.

That was the early spring cycle when I took advantage of

the surprisingly warm day to take a short bike ride around the city. The ride which revealed the city to be the polar opposite of the UK images I had been exposed to.

Upon return, I declared that now I was working from home and no longer commuting to work by bike, I would substitute that ride with a 30-minute lunchtime cycle along the coast for the benefit of both my body and my mind.

Ironically, as it turned out, that first whiff of spring air sparked a chain reaction which was actually detrimental to every element of health I had planned it to benefit. Both body and mind ended up taking a bit of a battering.

The first few weeks in April were innocent enough; the temperamental weather would see me both wrapped-up in layer upon layer, with a woolly hat pulled over my ears, pitting battle against and being buffered about by the city's formidable, reputable, and ceaseless winds. Alternatively, I'd be silkily gliding down a sun-splattered bike path through an ever-greening park. It felt both vascularly and psychologically invigorating. For now.

Meanwhile, my department manager, presumably with one genuinely caring eye on our well-being and another professionally demanding eye on our productivity, was keen to ensure her subordinates were all getting a regular dose of fresh air, screen breaks, and an opportunity to cyber socialise. She encouraged it, we had online lectures about the perils of inactivity. I have no doubts that her intentions were sincere and well-meaning, but she had no idea how the coronavirus was meddling with my psyche. She had no idea that what was 'well-meaning' to her, was akin to the actions of a psychopath, hellbent on my destruction with a bespoke insipidly evil-laced plan to both mentally torture and physically impair. She had given the thumbs-up for us to take care of ourselves, while at the same time – inadvertently or otherwise – giving me the thumbs-up to fuck myself up.

If my post-transplant motive for keeping as fit as possible stemmed from a fear of not being strong enough to face more surgery, then Covid 19, which reportedly had its crosshairs set on fat, wheezing, middle-aged men, resulted in me doubling down on my efforts. I might've looked the bespectacled bookworm as I tootled through town on Shep or Herman, but inside my head I was a commando, pumped up on Metallica, fist-bumps and adrenaline. I was in a tank. I was both 'shock' and 'awe'. My spirit was warfare, my body, more conscientious objector. Either way, I was on a mission.

All of a sudden, the kind of personal trainers who I'd previously overheard in the park, barking orders at huffing and puffing freshly divorced forty-somethings wearing spanking new Adidas tracksuits, had retreated to YouTube. There they plied their trade to a newly captivated (quite literally if you were in the UK and forcibly incarcerated by a lockdown) audience.

The world was being motivated to get in shape, and I was starting to question whether a 30-minute cycle ride was really enough. This city is pretty flat, after all, and when that wind was behind me, a sweat was nigh-on impossible to break in to.

I needed to up my game.

*****

There is perhaps something quite genuinely psychologically wrong with what helps inspire me to exercise. The net result of keeping fit, of course, is medically endorsed and encouraged, but how I get there, aside from my justified fear of dying at the hands of a surgeon, is questionable.

A few years before the Covid kick-off, there was a glut of sponsored photos on my Instagram feed posted by the pertest and prettiest pliable yoga 'hotties'. They were using the platform as a thinly disguised means of showing off their boobs, bums and fannies. Apparently, if you replace the words 'I want you to cum on my tits' with 'learn from yesterday, live for today, hope for tomorrow' alongside a photo of your face and glimpse of top-boob impossibly poking through your legs below your yoga-panted yet clearly defined labia, then the mysterious world of social media algorithms and poorly-paid internet slaves will wave your post through without question.

If the desired effect was to motivate, then in a roundabout and somewhat skewed manner, they achieved their goal. What really struck me was how these women, some of whom looked to have just as frail and weak a physique as I did, could perform feats of quite genuine strength. If they could do it, why couldn't I?

The headstand was definitely one of the favoured positions; images of women doing headstands on beaches and in the streets, legs akimbo or as straight as an arrow peppered my feed. It struck me that while I might be unsteady when standing the right way up, down to the fact that my sock-clad feet resembled the kind of makeshift weapon you might find being used in a prison riot, my head, was, to the best of my knowledge ... head shaped.

So out of nothing but pure spite for the world of the Beautiful Ables, I learned how to stand on my head. Stemming from an unbridled ire for the society around me, I went through the meditative breathing techniques and build-up exercises that the internet instructions regarded as a prerequisite for the move. It took a few months of wrath-induced gentle workouts and spite-filled yogic relaxation exercises, but I got there. It felt like vengeance, but at the same time gave me a sense of serene calmness every time I completed the exercise – more 'zen-geance' than 'vengeance', really.

*****

So in addition to the lunch cycle, I added a 30-minute routine of Pilates, push-ups, pull-ups, head standing and all sundry of non-weight-bearing exercises. Surely that was enough?

I've never been one to watch my weight. I have a team of medical staff who seem very happy to do that for me, although they are less concerned about fat, and more fretful of the return of water retention indicating my kidney is on the blink. Either way, I weigh about 66 kilos in the morning post poo, and about 67 before bed when poo from the day has reaccumulated. That puts me at the lower end of a normal BMI, and I was keen to maintain that equilibrium.

I've always had a certain sense of sensitivity about my weight, and in particular my skinny wrists. Friends' children love to compare their wrists with mine and shriek in glee, excitement, and disbelief when all the evidence before them suggests that they, despite being under the age of ten, are stronger than me. In addition, throughout my life I have been told by people, who should really know better, I need a good meal, I need fattening up, like I am a runt bullock they've promised to sell at market for slaughter.

Being born in 1973, I've come of age in classrooms where being fat, ginger, black, brown, Asian or a suspected homosexual were far more pressing on the Alpha Bullies' checklist of 'flaws'. I was under their radar, although it has left me being unquestionably sympathetic to people who bore the brunt of such micro and macro aggressions.

While my weight is not, and has never been, an obsession, I was keen that this new pandemic-themed lifestyle thrust upon me did not leave me further exposed to The Virus as a result of a steadily increasing BMI.

By about May 2020, I had been incrementally edging up my mileage for my daily cycle, and due to the ever-elongating days, I started to cycle in the evenings rather than lunchtime. It allowed for a longer and less frenzied bike ride, but at the same time increased the duration I was now static at my desk during office hours.

My university employer had upped its game in regard to our well-being, and academics from the sporty faculty started to share videos to help inspire us to get moving. Wherever I looked there was someone telling me to get off my bum. Despite all I was doing, I felt like I could do more.

Now the cycling had been confined to the evenings, I started to go on short walks at lunchtime. Nothing to upset my podiatrist, just a brief stroll, normally to the nearby recycling banks to dispose of the insane mountains of cardboard we were now accumulating due to the sudden spike in our home deliveries.

So a bit of exercise in the morning, a short walk at lunchtime, and an evening cycle. I was all set.

Until.

A friend had pointed out to me that in the most ubiquitous training tracking app, there was further motivation feature in the form of a challenge: if you could cycle the length of Sweden in the year 2020, you'd be sent a medal.

Now I am not the medal-seeking type, but something about the challenge appealed to me, and besides, I had been logging my mileage on the app anyway. I totted up the miles I had cycled so far, and calculated, now in June, that I was already halfway 'there'.

Having said that, the evening cycle was now being accompanied by my second favourite non-weight-bearing exercise, swimming. The waters around Sweden can be accurately described as 'bloody Baltic', chiefly because a lot of those waters are indeed part of the Baltic Sea.

Despite that, the newish UK trend of open-water swimming is rather more established in these parts, and a mid or post-workday dip is common practice. I found sea swimming exhausting, but it was added to the exercise regime all the same.

By early September, the end of the days were starting to dim, but I still had more than a third of Sweden left to cycle and I set the target of October the 25th by which to achieve this arbitrary goal. It was not a date plucked from thin air, but rather this was the day the clocks went back, an annual occurrence far more frustrating for me than anyone who thinks it is a bit sad when the days draw in. Every year that day marks the start of another lifestyle shift I have zero control over.

One of the complexities of my sort-of-saved sight is that my night vision is incredibly – and at times life-threateningly – poor. I try to avoid going out by myself. I need kerbs, lamp posts, puddles, cliff edges, and dodgy-looking people all pointed out to me. In addition, the fact that I have, effectively, tunnel vision makes me both a sitting mugging target and a danger unto myself. One thing I certainly don't do in dusky evenings is cycle at breakneck speed down an unlit coastal path.

The challenge might have stipulated the miles were to be completed by the end of 2020 for medal-awarding reasons, but for me, it was October 25th for life-saving reasons.

What followed was a full-on cycling frenzy. If it weren't for the fact that I was cycling a sit up and beg bike and wearing a corduroy jacket, and not hunched over a drop handlebar racer wearing Lycra, I might as well have been training for the Olympics.

I would cycle at lunch. I would cycle after work. And I'd clock every mile. Meanwhile, back at the office HQ, the powers that be were, unbeknown to me, plotting. Just as I was closing in on my goal, a notification from the HR department, cheered on by my manager, was dispatched. The missive revealed a thinly veiled ploy to keep the 2,000 or so members of staff from taking unnecessary sick days. It read:

On October 26, a five-week activity challenge starts. By logging all your physical activities, from a lunch stroll to gardening to marathon training or Zumba session, you can participate and challenge other teams.

You will be using an app to log your activity and follow your team members and cheer them on during the challenge. Your activities will automatically be converted into points.

So quite literally the day after my own personal challenge was set to come to a grand anticlimactic close, another five weeks of gladiatorial one-upmanship was due to commence.

Come October 25th I was broken and saddle sore. My feet seemed unharmed, but they ached from the endless pedal stress; either way, the challenge had been achieved. I had cycled the length of Sweden in 80 cycles. Obviously if I had actually cycled from the southern tip to the northernmost icy end, I would have chanced upon rivers, mountains, forests, and the Arctic Circle, but I think the fact that I cycled it on an 85-year-old bike with no gears, at least in part, made up for the geographical pancake nature of where I live.

Sweden is 978 miles long, and as I crossed the imaginary finishing tape, I had amassed 1001.86 miles. As a point of reference, the longest country in the world is Chile, which is 2,653 miles, and the oft-trod Land's End at the bottom of England to Scotland's John O'Groats, is 603 miles.

I had challenged myself and I had won, but what came next piqued my post-transplant raison d'être – compete against The Ables and beat them at their own games. I can't say the cycle hadn't left me a little jaded and in need of some rest and recuperation after its frenzied conclusion, but the timing of this new challenge was out of my hands. I had to hit the ground running. Well, cycling at least.

It worked like this: to take part, you downloaded an app where teams of six could be registered. Every time an activity was logged, the app would award points based on the duration and intensity of the exercise. The HR department set a minimum number of points for each individual to achieve within a given week; all team members had to reach that bare minimum to 'successfully' complete the week. In the app, there was also a list which ranked every individual irrespective of teams with the number one spot being reserved for the most active participant – this chart was in a constant state of flux, as individuals from across the workforce logged their activities throughout the day.

Not the worst initiative our HR department could've come up with to nudge an unknown number of individuals who, from behind working-from-home closed doors, were piling on the pounds having possibly forgone their own daily cycle to the office. And of course, the manager of our department could relax, safe in the knowledge that ample opportunity and time had been granted to her staff to exercise and prevent any further physical and mental degradation that the pandemic could incur. If this, indeed, was an underhand ploy to rid me from the payroll, then she now had willing accomplices, or at the very least, the HR department to blame.

I set to it the morning after having completed my length-of-Sweden cycle. And I started it with another bike ride. Flexi-working hours allowed me to get to my desk around ten in the morning, so plenty of time to squeeze in a 15-mile cycle. I immediately registered the ride and was delighted to see that not only had I smashed the weekly HR-set target, but I was also in the number one position out of the several hundred colleagues who had already chosen to participate.

For them, I was just another name on the list. Some had met me, some hadn't. But I see all those names as The Ables (although statistically speaking, I doubt they all were); these people were not aware of the physical ailments I had to overcome before I could compete on their level. And I wasn't just competing – I was winning. This had nothing to do with teams anymore. This had nothing to do with fresh air and screen breaks. This was a battle – me against them – and two hours after the challenge started, I had thrown down the gauntlet. I'm not sure how obsessively people were monitoring the overall chart section, but my name sitting there at the top of the list belied a motive I feel like I have no control over – be better at everything than anyone else.

*****

I am not entirely sure where my competitive streak, which feels more like a competitive gorge at times, comes from, but it is deeply entrenched. Perhaps it is the fact that I am the youngest of two brothers. Forever in the shadow of an elder, it is the youngest son's duty to upstage the Big Brother. If I was gonna have to wear his hand-me-downs, then surely I'd try to achieve more in those patched-up, brown corduroy trousers than he ever did.

In reality, between me and my brother, while at times I've indubitably been the shouty, cry-y, door slam-y, emotive, attention-demanding one, there never felt like there was any competition between us. We've always competed on very different playing fields.

On a physical level, there is no way I could beat my brother, even before my disabilities kicked in. He is not only physically stronger but also far more adventurous and much sportier. I thought 'circuit training' was just running round the gym in circles until he explained otherwise. He hikes, he runs, he gyms, he fences, he has been on Arctic expeditions and has trekked through perilous mountain ranges and dangerous deserts. I could never compete against him, even if I felt genetically bound to do so. I once borrowed his camping stove to use at a music festival; I do recall a pang of guilt as I sparked up a joint from what I knew to be a pretty pricey bit of kit. I guess that is how we differ.

Of course there was also my father. He was a regimented and ordered man who had been parented by a strict private prep school, a harsh boarding school and then the Royal Air Force. The kind of man who, after a hard week's work as a sales manager, would take off his work tie and slip into something more comfortable – a weekend tie. I am sure I have a recollection of him wearing silk-knit neckwear as he mowed the lawn.

He was a man who enjoyed 'bloody good walks' and swimming. In fact, the older he got, the more besotted he became with the sea and swimming in it. Upon the demise of his relationship with my mother, he relocated to the southern coast of Britain where he found a flat so close to the English Channel that he could navigate the 30-metre walk from his front door to the perma-chilled ebbing surf without having to put his contact lenses in.

Towards the end of his life, he chose the bargain-basement option of circumnavigating the globe as the sole paying guest on a working cargo ship. I never saw a photo of that boat, but the decks were not so high as to prevent him from throwing himself overboard every time the captain notified the crew they were now entering a new sea. As patience for my father's foolhardiness dwindled, and the novelty wore off, the crew had to make a point of preventing him from this apparently suicidal desire. Fishing him out was slowing the progress of their main task – delivering stuff to schedule. If perhaps you had a late parcel delivery sometime between 2000 and 2001, it might very well be because the shipping process was delayed by a crew of sailors yanking my dad out of the South China Sea.

Then there's mum. Speaking subjectively, of course, she has always seemed to me, better than anyone else's mum. I recall being away for a week-long cub camp when I was nine years old. Our cub scout leader (Akela) asked me to console a friend of mine who was suffering from homesickness. I have never thought of myself as an empathic or motivating kind of person, and perhaps what I said to this boy, sobbing about missing his mother, was an early indication of this fact. I am not sure what the Akela wanted me to say or what my friend wanted to hear, but what he got was this: 'You shouldn't miss your mum. I don't miss mine, and she's loads better than yours'.

The older I got, the more objective my understanding became of how good my mum is at stuff. To this very day, she likes to remind me of how my friends would knock on our door and ask her if she wanted to come out and play, with me being an afterthought. She's a natural at everything she turns her hand to. She took up archery as a 40th birthday present to herself, and now her spare room is littered with medals and trophies and bits of old bows. She's always the social secretary at every place she has ever worked, organising days out not just out of a desire to make sure people felt bonded but also because she just likes to do stuff. For as long as I can remember, she has been lending her hand to a parish news magazine which keeps two villages up to date on when the next fete is (with an accompanying plea for volunteers to staff the tombola stall), and classified ads normally offering dog-walking and babysitting services (a section I imagine has grown ten-fold with pandemic-propelled job losses). The magazine was never meant to be a business enterprise, but from the outset, my mother changed paper suppliers, mercilessly haggled with printers and now the magazine makes a tidy profit which can be ploughed back into the community.

That's my mum: popular, sociable, and competitive. If I was competing against her, I'd hate her, but she is normally, although not exclusively, on my side.

She was, but no longer is, thanks to being 'woked' by my incessant castigation, a bit of a fat-shamer. If you were under 30, didn't have the honed body of an Olympic athlete or a Cosmopolitan model and were exposing even the slightest bit of flabby midriff, bum, or beer belly, she'd pass comment. This would normally happen when I was a passenger in her car as we drove through the traffic-calmed centre of her local town. I would like to say it was under her breath, but I was paranoid it was audible to the subject of the taunt, particularly as such comments were more likely to be made during the summer months when the car windows were down and the level of skin on show was at its highest.

So that's my family for you. Not overtly sporty, but certainly my upbringing was one that valued physical prowess, regimented dedication, lunacy, inherent skill, and a smidge of fat shaming. What chance did I have of not growing up with a fierce, competitive streak and a desire to keep my skinny frame just that, skinny?

*****

Perhaps the fact that I had become accustomed to cycling morning, noon, and summer night meant I could just carry on with what I had already started, bar the now ever-shortening night slot. It certainly felt like adequate exercise, and seeing that the first ride I completed was enough for me to reach the weekly target and put me in the number one spot, this challenge was a shoo-in, surely?

As it turned out, no.

I had a nemesis. A Swedish nemesis.

A Nemesisson.

Just a bloke who worked for the same institution as I, in reality, but in my mind, he was the apex of The Ables. When I checked later on that first day of the challenge to ensure my top spot was still secure, I saw, to my absolute horror, I had been usurped from my perch by a name I was not familiar with. The man, AKA the Nemesisson, who was to become my sworn app-based enemy for the next five weeks.

He had not just totalled my point tally but smashed it. Alongside Nemesisson, I could see that there would be a constant fight for pole position from a number of competitors. People had started to take this seriously. No matter how insistent HR and various managers were that this was just a gentle way to get us moving, it was clearly obvious this was being treated as a full-on challenge of Hunger Games proportions.

Bring. It. On.

While it was the wintery end of October, I was still open water swimming. Added to that was, of course, my daily workout routine and walk. It was hard to work out how it could be feasible to fit any more exercise in the day without compromising my work duties, but Nemesisson was somehow managing it.

Days rolled into weeks, and we continued to tussle for

the top spot – well I did, he was probably completely oblivious to his determined competitor (me). While I often temporarily won the battle, he was winning the war. His weekly point score was ebbing further and further out of reach.

But fortune favours the … foolhardy. I had long since booked a week off to use up holiday time that would otherwise have been spent to travel to the now-out-of-bounds UK. I probably should have used the week to relax, take my mind off work, off the ever-present threat of death and disease which plagued my subconscious as much as it was plaguing the world around me. But no, there were points to be scored, and now there were no work hours to distract me from catching up with Nemesisson's tally.

I had noticed a Facebook advert posted by a German woman who lived in my city who was offering handstand lessons. If I could already stand on my head, then how hard could standing on my hands be? Hands are a lot more like feet than heads, after all. I signed up.

What followed were two four-hour sessions which were hosted in an outdoor gym. And when I say 'gym', what I actually mean is a clearing in a forested bit of park. It was just me and her. I made her aware of my physical limitations, told her how easily my feet would break if I crash-landed onto them, and how my core had been split in two and would never quite be the same again. She ably avoided my troubled spots and instead exploited what was left. What had not been previously broken or rendered by surgery, she pushed to the brink.

Every sinew in my body ached for the days that followed those sessions. Turns out you need to strengthen more than just hands to do a handstand. Still, it was a massive point boost to my tally.

It was Week 3 of the 5-week challenge. I could feel my muscles were sore, but that was to be expected. I also could feel my groin aching, but that's what comes of spending endless hours on an 85-year-old saddle. Still, something else wasn't right.

I know my body well. I know when my blood pressure is low, high, or ebbing in either direction. I know if the glucose levels in my blood are high just by how it oozes from a lanceted fingertip. I know when there is too much iron in my system just by the colour of my poo. I know when I have overhydrated and my electrolytes are depleting by just a whiff of wee. I know my body, and I knew something was amiss.

There are certain things I can rule out with bits of medical equipment I have amassed over the years. My blood pressure was fine, my blood sugars were fine, my poo smelled like poo, and my wee smelled like wee.

But wait, there was something I had not checked, something I hardly ever check.

Due to my now constant weight, the bathroom scales have been largely untouched. For the sake of ruling it out, I checked. And there it was. Now, instead of having a BMI at the lower end of normal, I had a BMI at the upper end of underweight. What was I doing to myself?

But the challenge beckoned, and my competitive streak was not going anywhere fast. And if it was going to go somewhere fast, you can bet I'd try to catch it up and beat it – that being part of the problem with competitive streaks. The only thing I could do was take in more calories, and seeing as I might potentially add to my paltry muscles with all the exercise, some additional protein to boot.

This is what the innocent motivational challenge had

made me. I doubled my complex carbohydrates at breakfast by making my porridge with an extra scoop of oats.
I'd eat three eggs instead of two, and I'd eat pastries with
guilt-free gluttony for quick fix bursts of glucose.

But ultimately, there was nothing I could do. My unwitting nemesis extended his lead. I did a 40-mile ride as my
last hurrah, a desperate bid to claw myself into the top 10,
but nothing, nothing could get me there.

Weeks later, the HR dispatched a congratulatory email to all
those involved. It was like poking an open wound and I, better
than most, know what that feels like. Predictably, Nemesisson was named as the highest achieving participant. Within the mail were the Top 10 individuals. My name was not
among them. I tried to compete with The Ables and failed.

It hurt my pride, knowing that even though I 'walk
among them', I am not capable of the same physical feats.
It wasn't as if the Top 10 was made up of the fresh-faced
gym bunnies of the workforce. Even my manager (whose
age began with '5' as opposed to mine which started with
a '4') was ranked in fifth position, and I hadn't noticed her
chugging energy drinks during our departmental Zoom
meetings, and I don't think she took time off to coincide
with the demands of the challenge.

By the time that email had arrived, my weight was back
to normal, the muscle pains had subsided, and I was back
to my regular doses of porridge and egg intake. The only
real lasting scar was a psychological one. I might feel like
an Olympian when I compete against myself, but when I
am pitted against The Ables, I fall at the first hurdle.

I can only be as fit as this body allows, and all I could really hope for is that it would be fit enough to overcome the
challenges this pandemic would throw at me.

Chapter 8
My least favourite eye appointment, ever

I never really got to know my granny – down to the peculiar machinations of that particular side of the family – but I did know she had cataracts. As did her son, my dad, although he didn't know his own mother that well either.

'Wait until I've put my eyes in', was a cry I frequently heard as a child as he did daily battle with his contact lenses. It was the response I often received whenever I nagged him about driving me to my primary school in a neighbouring village. Sometimes friends would overhear it, prompting anything from curious *WTF*?-raised eyebrows to genuine fear that my dad was in an adjacent room screwing in some eyeballs – that he kept in a glass of water overnight on his bedside set of drawers – into empty, bloodied, ocular sockets.

I recall him having a number of surgeries to correct his vision, but I was too young to question why, or join any dots between his hospital stays and his mum's habit of hammering her shins into bits of clearly visible furniture when she graced us with her presence.

In his early twenties, during his short stint in the Royal Air Force, my father had participated in the sport of boxing; that particular armed service, bafflingly, encourage such an activity. Why it would proffer up pilots to repeatedly biff each other in the face when the participating pugilists' careers depended on 20/20 vision perhaps says it all about an organisation which has considered 'carpet bombing' and 'drone strikes' as viable solutions to an in-box query from the Foreign Office.

It was the barbarism of boxing which floored both my dad and his RAF career. During a mis-matched fight, he was punched into a coma by a man twice his weight and height; with the same punch, both his retinas simultaneously detached. He had only just passed his pilot exams. Now, facing a career behind a desk, he demobbed and quit. Instead of using his eyes for a high-octane career flying jet fighters, he used them to navigate a company car as a mediocrely paid sales manager for a building supplies firm. The cataracts in both eyes that he also later suffered from were a develop-one-get-one-free hereditary hand-me-down from his mother.

Despite all the genetic evidence laid out before me, it came as quite a shock when, at the age of nineteen, the optician I had known since I was a kid informed me I too had cataracts in both eyes. Out of all the reactions I could have instinctively been overwhelmed by upon hearing such news, the one I could never have predicted was, embarrassment. Cataracts were for blue-rinsed and Brylcreemed geriatrics, not a mop-haired indie kid – an identity my formative years were morphing me into. At the time, I was happy wigging-out to Blur, not so happy seeing through a blur.

I never told my dad; this was not the kind of thing I wanted to bond over. I don't recall telling anyone, in fact, other than my mother who had driven me to the appointment. This all happened while I was at university, before I had learned how to drive, before I had really learned how to live.

It's hard to put such news to the back of your mind, particularly as – anatomically – 'the back of your mind' is very close to where your optical nerves end. It left me feeling insecure, quite genuinely uncertain about whether I was ever getting the 'full picture', that there was something I might have been missing, the subtleties of life. The condition, in reality, bore no real significance, and it wasn't hard to keep it under the radar. The closest I got to being rumbled was when I took my driving test at the age of 23. I knew before I'd even get to sit in the driving seat beside the examiner that I would have the 'minor detail' of a nonchalant eye test. The kind casually performed by the man, in this case, pointing to a car some 20 metres away and asking me to read the number plate. It was this, and not the prospect of failure or the embarrassment of three-point turning over a toddler who had chased their ball into a cul-de-sac, that kept me fretting the night before the test.

On the day, the sun shone in my favour; he pointed to a random car parked down the road, and I ably read the plate. Had he turned around and pointed to a vehicle the other way down the same street, a car parked in the shadows, he probably would have been met with the response, 'What car?'. Still, once I had passed the test, I was far more in control of the roads I chose to travel down. Instinctively, it made me a nervous driver, but at the same time, a safer one – no toddlers died when I was behind the wheel ... that I ever felt the bone-crunching bump of, anyway.

FOR THE (MEDICAL) RECORD

Some people live in ivory towers, but not my gran. After the death of her spouse, she lived in an ivory apartment, or rather an apartment liberally scattered with ornamentally carved elephant tusks. I am assured by people who knew her that she was a popular, fun-loving and sociable character, which might very well have been the case, but the history books in which she is a footnote, are drenched in blood, and she was definitely on the side of the aggressors who did the blood spilling.

Both she and her husband were the products of the spoils of empire building. With his job, they jaunted around the world for decades – keeping pretty much exclusively to the bits of the map deemed cordial or colonialised.

My father was dragged from pillar to outpost before, at the age of eight, he was thrust into the British private education system, the bill for which was footed by his dad's employer. During the lion's share of his education, he saw his parents every four years and, as an adult, did not look back upon this time with any iota of fondness.

That side of the family were old-school posh shitbags. My dad's sibling continued the tradition by managing a cocoa plantation farm in West Africa, perhaps you've heard of it? It's called 'Ghana', more of a country to you and I. One of dad's cousins was the Tory MP, Ian Grist, who went into politics after a quick working tour of the fast-crumbling empire.

One might expect that with such privilege comes pots of cash and a castle, but nothing could be further from the truth. The reality was, any family fortune was lost by my great grandparents with bungled business deals, a bourgeois lifestyle and staggeringly bad bets. Something I am, with the benefit of education, truly glad of – a blood money-funded life of privilege is not a life for me.

But that history left its mark on my dad, and subsequently also me. My dad was a man steeped in the ways and mannerisms of the upper-middle classes. He spoke 'the Queen's English', he could tie a Windsor knot without a second thought or YouTube tutorial, and he jokingly referred to the rest of the family as heathens for refusing to attend church. He didn't like me and my brother watching Grange Hill in fear I'd pick up a slangy north London accent, he didn't like us watching ITV, for that matter, as it just smacked of crassness in his – admittedly shitty – eyes. He was conservative with a big and a little 'c'. He was queen, country, and the BBC through and through. But he was also a humbly paid sales manager, with no education beyond a modern-day GCSE level equivalent, who drove around the southeast of England flogging nuts and bolts to building contractors.

I remember once, at my primary school gates, some friends pointing out how my dad looked down his nose while he drove. Of course 'looking down one's nose' is a stereotype of the aloof and snooty, and there was my dad, who might have been mistaken for being both of those things, actually doing it.

I never really thought anything of it until decades later, and some years after I passed my driving test. As the cataracts did their worst, I found myself increasingly flipping down the sun visor to protect myself from the sun's glare. That, on occasion, mystified passengers who were bemused by why I'd need to do such a thing. But cataracts cause light sensitivity, so towards the end of my driving days I kept the sun visor down. I also found that if I raised my head and looked down my nose, it'd increase what I could see and the clarity by which I could see it. Exactly like my dad had done.

Now, in my late 40s, I can see how various disabilities have encroached on my behaviour and, in a sense, re-shaped my identity. For example, thanks to my deformed ankle bones, my days of being able to run have been rendered over, no matter the distance. But instead of not being able to run to catch a bus, I've become the kind of person who simply doesn't run for buses ('there is not a bus in the world worth running for, my dear.'). In theory, I have no grudge against busy bars where one needs to jostle for service, but such venues often mean you end up standing or meeting friends in dimly lit, crowded corners – my eyes and feet allow for neither. Restaurants and 'more civilised establishments' are, by default, far more accessible venues. I do my best to be early when meeting friends in a public space or venue, that way they have to find me (which they can do using the medium of 'sight'), as opposed to me accidentally walking right past them (which I usually do using the medium of sight loss). So, now I've become the type of person who avoids public transport (for myriad health reasons), prefers quieter and more serene surrounds, and is always punctual. Add to that my perma-home counties accent, and I can appear like a proper stuck-up twat. Which I ain't.

When these things become your lived experiences, empathy and understanding become second nature. If I am being held up in a supermarket queue by someone faffing around with their wallet or purse, I don't assume 'inconsideration', I think, 'Are they having a panic attack?' or 'Do they have Parkinson's disease?'. Is the person who refuses to move out of the way when walking down a pavement a selfish prick, or do they have OCD – you don't honestly know, do you?

*****

From around 2000 to 2002, my job as an agency news reporter forced me to both drive at odd hours and file stories on my laptop on the hoof. It was before GPS was really accessible for people on piss-poor incomes, and I'd find myself lost down country lanes in the back of beyond, using a keyring torch to locate the address of the door to be knocked in a dog-eared A-Z street map with alarmingly frequency. Either that or sitting on courthouse steps in the baking heat with a coat slung over my head to keep the glare from my screen as I furiously sent copy down the wires.

I was now in my late twenties, and my optician considered my case a matter of urgency. As someone whose age betrayed their ailment, I was fast-tracked up the waiting list. My eyesight was restored by means of two cataract operations. My life reset, I was amazed by how much I could now see, the ophthalmologists, however, were less impressed.

They had found scarring at the back of my eye, and it was then that I was referred to Doctor 'if-you-get-on-that-plane-to-LA-you-will-go-blind' Fleet. I am not sure quite what distinguishes the title of 'professor', as in Professor Mike Edmonds (the man who had saved my life and feet), from the title of 'doctor' as in, Doctor 'I'll-nonchalantly-destroy-your-life' Fleet, but I suspect the latter bunked off her bedside manner lectures and spent the time instead using the sun to burn ants through her newly acquired set of optical lenses. I am not questioning her professionalism in the slightest, but she had the manner of Kathy Bates' character in the horror film *Misery*. She was the one who prescribed the numerous bouts of laser treatment to reduce the scarring and minimise the risk of a potential bleed. That procedure meant me putting on a massive pair of goggles, which kept my eyes hydrated, while Fleet, or one of her cohorts, effectively played space invaders with the back of my retinas. Each zap was a permanent burn, and the peripheral vision I now live with, and my inability to see colours, is a side effect of this treatment.

I assume they did everything they could, or maybe they were just shit at space invaders, whatever, it was towards the end of 2002 that the blood started to leak through the scarring, and it was then that I went blind in one eye mid-dinner party.

'We're going to have to send you to the big guns', was all a defeated Deborah could tell me, as she crushed my Los Angeles dreams and my nan (my mum's mum, who I was infinitely closer to than my dad's mum) gently passed away in a nearby wing of the hospital.

FOR THE (MEDICAL) RECORD

You've probably pondered what it is like to be or go blind, possibly sparked by a schoolyard debate over which sense you'd least like to lose or trying to wrap your head around the fact that some people don't even understand the concept of colour.

What do you think would frustrate you the most? Not seeing your family and friends, or not being able to take a selfie? Never being able to binge watch Netflix again? The more you start to consider the gradual or sudden loss of your vision, the more the miseries pile up.

Personally, I can list a steady stream of frustrations, including such trivialities as not knowing when an art-house movie flicks between black and white to colour in order to convey an emotion. The glorious reality is, however, I can see well enough to sit at a computer and type. So sitting at a computer and typing is what I've made my life.

I am unquestionably lucky to have a job, a job which brings me into contact with many people. I also live in a small and friendly apartment block. Everyone I work with and live among seems jolly, approachable and chatty.

But here's the thing: I probably (don't) see these people in the supermarket, in the streets, even in the elevators at work. They are there. It's just that I don't see them.

For all intents and purposes, I am ignoring them. I am blanking them. Because the frustrations you list when considering sight loss rarely include embarrassment.

Inevitably many sufferers of sight loss will have overlapping 'top frustration', but the nuances of sight loss are many and may not be as apparent or as obvious as you would consider.

As someone who has a job and doesn't require a white stick, I know I am, relatively, more blessed than cursed, but I am sure in my wake I've unwittingly caused offence as I inadvertently snub acquaintances. It pains the inherent polite nature at my core knowing that I have no idea of how many people I have caused mild-mannered offence to.

I now find myself paralysed by the prospect of saying hello to a complete stranger because my optical nerves are telling my brain they are my closest colleague. I stare at the floor as I shuffle around stores in fear I'll lock eyes with the chap who may or may not be the neighbour who only that morning I had held the communal door open for.

As it stands: two women I work with look like my mother-in-law, three guys who live in my apartment block look like they were separated at birth, I have to second-glance every time I see my brother in the work elevator (and he doesn't even live in this country), and one woman who has worked in my office for two weeks looks the absolute spit of another woman who has been there for two years.

I often have to identify people by situation, by voice, by gait, by fashion statements, but there are times I quite genuinely do not approach people in fear I make a fool of myself.

Such a disability naturally brings with it a sense of vulnerability. Combine that with the fact that my limited vision forces me to behave in a way that contradicts my true polite and gregarious nature, and you can perhaps start to understand the further frustrations of the partially sighted.

*****

So, off to the 'big guns' it was for me. Now, I am no fan of guns of any size to be honest, but the surgeon I was referred to who would now be calling 'the shots' was, firstly, not that 'big', and secondly, armed only with a scalpel – something he brandished with some aplomb, if my experiences with him were anything to go by.

Fleet had scared the bejesus out of me. I was petrified

as to what the big gun, or Mr Martin Snead as he is more commonly referred to as, would do to me. On his first inspection, I was expecting him to pull back and tell me my eyes were fucked and the next step would be to get measured for glass eyeballs. What he actually said, however, in a comforting and reassuring voice which plucked my nerve-wracked psyche from the pits of despair, was 'Yes, I think we can sort this out'.

Years later, the last words he ever said to me – once again as he pulled back from an eye inspection – seemingly having no awareness of how much I wanted to hug him and break down in tears of relief – were 'Yes, I think we are done with you now'.

It did take four surgeries between 2004 and 2011, a multitude of overnight hospital stays and more appointments than you can shake a white cane at, but we, or rather Snead and his team, got there.

And 'there' I stayed, at least in regard to the stability of my retinas, which have remained as he left them ever since his last scalpel-tinkering. Although one meaning of the word 'there' did change – where 'there' actually was. My eye care, along with all my other ailment care, was transferred into the capable hands of the Swedish healthcare system. To this day, and from November 2011 when I moved to Sweden, my eyes are checked once a year, always by a different ophthalmologist, and I can guarantee that after they roll back on their specially designed eye examination chairs, they'll exclaim, 'Wow, someone has been busy in there!' or words to that effect.

Since my move to 'there' – a country I now refer to as 'here', in addition to the annual eye tests, I have an appointment with my transplant consultant every three months, *that* routine blood test once a month, and my feet are checked on an ad hoc basis varying from very hoc, when a sore mysteriously appears on one of my lumps, to not so hoc, when the podiatrist just gives me what amounts to a medical-grade pedicure.

While my consultants and carers have chopped and changed since my 'big' surgery and subsequent move to Sweden, I have found myself becoming increasingly trusting and familiar with, in particular, my transplant consultant and my foot specialist (known not-to-her-knowledge as 'the Foot Lady'). I can't say that the smell of hospitals and clinics don't evoke depressing memories, but I rarely stress when I turn up at the hospital for a routine appointment. While any part of my anatomy might spin out of control with no fair warning, years of stable results and checks have given me some sense of comfort that both myself and my care partners are collaborating well.

Well, that was the case up until March 2020.

Face masks might have been a bang-on trend in Bangkok airport when we returned from Thailand, but in Sweden there was only a certain ilk who could be seen wearing them: 'You bought "Tinfoil hat in size medium", people who looked at this item also looked at "5 disposable face masks" – buy together for €15'. They were still so rare that, while the rest of Europe looked like they were off to collect forensics from a crime scene in a disused asbestos factory, in Sweden, if you saw someone wearing one as you cycled to work, then for many who still 'braved' the office, they were probably a good conversation starter in the elevator.

Personally, I was in two minds from the start. My Facebook timeline was filling up with sponsored face mask adverts, each clamouring to claim theirs was the most breathable and reusable; often, I noted, seldom stating how effective they were. Soon, those adverts were punctuated by selfies of UK friends gurning behind an array of homemade or novelty face coverings – even some of my anti-selfie friends were at it, possibly on the grounds that covering half your face takes decades off you.

At this time, the only other apartment on the same floor as ourselves had been sold. We lamented the fact that its previous tenant had relocated, not on the grounds that we were on cup-of-sugar-borrowing good terms with him but rather, based on the scant evidence we had, that he was single, middle-aged, quiet, and hardly ever in. My heart sank when I spied through our peephole a couple in their thirties carting in moving boxes. He was wearing a hoodie. I could see a guitar. They had a dog. Fuck. I couldn't see her, but I could hear her; they were speaking English, but she had an accent, a Chinese accent.

I couldn't recall the last time I had read or watched anything about China without an accompanying image or footage of a bat, someone drinking a cup of tea with a tentacle poking out of it, or a photo of a recently deceased whistle-blowing doctor. If China's reputation comes out of this unscathed, I imagine Tiananmen Square statues of the future will be of the government's PR department's employees.

I wasn't too sure whether I should hastily nail their front door shut with them inside, cordon the flat off with hazard tape and hold my breath every time I was in the lobby, or suggest we meet for a drink to introduce ourselves. In the end, I went for the latter.

As it turned out, Brandy, the Chinese woman in question, had not long returned from visiting her motherland for the super-spreader event of the century, Chinese New Year, 2020. Upon her return, her husband, Will, had quarantined himself away for two weeks, possibly perusing the IKEA website and hoping that his wife would be fine, and he'd need to order a double rather than a single bed for the apartment they were soon to move into.

We were all newbies to socialising mid-plague and considered 'ours' and 'theirs' bowls of peanuts as the ultimate precaution to prevent infection. It came out, during our first of now many get-togethers, that when Brandy visited her family home, her parents had insisted she was only to wear 'made in China' face masks upon her return to Sweden; crappy European-manufactured ones were clearly not up to scratch. I mentioned that I was soon to have my first blood test in a pandemic, and that I was considering buying some masks. The next day, I found a bag of China's finest paper face masks in our post box. I was strangely reassured by the fact that I'd be wearing a piece of protective garb produced by the country which had, as it then stood, the upper hand in its fight against the virus. As it transpired, these neighbours have proved to be better than the last – in addition, I have never heard their dog bark, or Will play the guitar.

So now it was me who was one of the face mask wearing 'ilk'. While they had limited the numbers who could wait for a blood test, I was the only one wearing a mask. I actually felt guilty when the phlebotomist drew my blood. She was a frontline worker, and I was more 'protected' than she was. On top of that, at least the blood-taking process does afford one the luxury of looking away and your face turned from unmasked mouths and noses:

Q: 'Why are you looking away, are you afraid of needles?'

A: 'No, I am afraid you might kill me'.

The next appointment, in April, was with my foot specialist. She saw me and my familiar partially lumbering gait amble towards the treatment room and scurried off. I was once again sporting a China-supplied face mask, and her policy was, if the patient wore one, so would she, although she did joke that the very nature of her feet-inspecting job would keep her from me by at least two metres – I'm 183cm tall and her arms are definitely longer than 17cm.

My transplant appointments were now conducted by phone, as all the doctor really needed were my blood tests to assess my health. By the time the UK had come out of its first lockdown in June 2020, I had still not seen any healthcare provider in Sweden other than Foot Lady, who possibly only ever wore a face mask in my presence. Nor, for that matter, had I seen any friend or colleague wear one. The health boffs who were governing Sweden's pandemic response never wore them either and still seemed highly sceptical of their benefits.

So, despite my best-laid plans to keep myself safe, it was, ironically, only when I went to see some of the people who were there to take care of me that I felt most exposed. Anyone who has been a serial in-patient will know you leave your pride at the hospital door, where your care is duly handed over to medical professionals.

If and when you are lucky enough to be discharged, your care is only partially handed back to you. What once was all yours, is now a shared responsibility. You find yourself bound by an unwritten contract citing that your care is now the responsibility of both you and your healthcare providers.

While I did my utmost to keep my side of the 'care contract', the Swedish healthcare systems were, for the greater part of 2020, in breach of theirs. I knew better than to trust politicians, but now my faith in professors was also in doubt. It was hard for me to fathom why the 'they're better than nothing' logic, which prevailed in the UK face mask debate, would trump Sweden's 'they'll give people a false sense of security and people won't use them correctly anyway' logic. The Swedish argument might very well be the case, but for vulnerable people having to regularly visit places which, by their very purpose, are chock-a-block with the sick and the snotty, it seemed as if I was more attentive to this 'care contract' than my Swedish partners.

It wasn't just the professors and politicians who kept face masks off faces, Sweden no doubt suffered as a result of its limited purchasing power in the Great PPE Rush of Spring 2020. But one autumn day, as I rolled up my sleeve for my monthly bloodletting, I found, for the first time, the face of the nurse was obscured by both a visor and a face mask, although another nurse attending a patient just metres away from me was wearing neither. Meanwhile, in the UK, you would not have looked out of place doing your weekly shop in a hazmat suit.

To me, it felt like a lottery. I had no idea what level of protection I'd get every time I walked through a hospital door. And there was one appointment which weighed heavily on my mind – my annual eye examination.

There's no way around it. For a doctor to thoroughly check the backs of my eyes, they need to stare at me intently, nose to nose, for up to ten minutes. It can feel rather awkward. I'm just not comfortable with that level of eye contact, but I pride myself on being a good patient, so I persevere. Of course, I could have sacked off the appointment, but what if something was awry? What if the stability that Snead the Surgeon had established was starting to wobble?

If there was one individual outlier who rallied against the country now deemed a global outlier, it was my friend Christine. She's the acceptable face of survivalism – she might've been prepping for the worst, but among her hoard of food, water, and, I kid you not, an oxygen concentration device, there was not an AK-47 or Rambo knife in sight. She wasn't erring on the side of caution but rather being cautious of veering away from precaution. It was time to upgrade from Chinese face masks, and who better to ask about the best on the market? During a heavily sterilised outside exchange (possibly with the wind blowing in her favour, I'd wager), she handed me, I was assured, the most effective mask to keep the bugs at bay.

The next day at the hospital, I was relieved to see that while the reception staff were not wearing masks, the first nurse I saw, was. Although, as it transpired, it was all a bit of a 'farce mask'. For one of the tests, I had to take the mask off in order to get close enough to the equipment. All the other medical staff I saw walking past were not wearing one. I'd never felt so exposed.

For the next few days, I just full-on isolated myself to be sure I was okay. I can only speak from what I observed, but it did seem that by mid-October guidance was given to medical staff to don the necessaries when they were within a two-metre radius of the patient. On numerous occasions I was in a smallish consulting room talking to an unmasked specialist, only for them to PPE-up when it was time to encroach on my personal space.

I had previously been relishing the freedom I had on

this side of the North Sea, but I was increasingly jealous of the cotton wool my vulnerable friends in the UK were being swaddled in.

I never missed my dad's mother, the granny I barely knew, but I sure was starting to miss my UK nanny ... state.

Chapter 9
The problem with a fully-functioning welfare state

So, you are about to embark on the 'cock chapter'. This fair warning is not meant in any shape or form as page-turning clickbait but rather to alert you to the fact that it contains graphic descriptions of a number of eye-watering traumas and batterings my genitalia suffered as a result of my ill health. The chapter also contains vivid recounts of a sexual nature and wanking references. It is not intended to be gratuitous, and I consider it an essential part of the narrative. If you are of the male persuasion and wince and recoil at even the thought of catching your foreskin in your trouser zipper, don't say I didn't warn you.

Here we go ...

It is true to say that between 2009 and 2010, more people had tugged on my willy than in the previous twenty-plus years of serial monogamist sexual activity. In fact, while numbers are blurry, it could be true that more people grappled with my willy in the first 24 hours I was in Sweden than during my span of post-virginity-losing vanilla-rising with the opposite sex.

There is no question about it, I am intimate – on so many levels – with both the UK's National Health Service and the Swedish Health Authorities. The NHS had cared for me from the cradle to one foot in the grave; in fact, they had yoinked me from that premature grave which, at the age of 37, when my transplant surgery was carried out, was too soon after the cradle-end of their duties. They had re-plumbed me with the new organs, patched me up and, on my own request just over a year later, forwarded my medical history, perhaps requiring their own shipping container, to the Swedes.

Is there a better way to demonstrate 'intimacy', at least in my prudish-English mind, than with a willy story? And the 'joy' of this particular willy story, is that of its cross-border nature. It is a true tale of collaboration, which took place when the reality of an EU referendum was nothing more than a splodgy mess Nigel Farage found soiling his bed sheets after waking from an 'early withdrawal' wet dream.

*****

Back in 2009, the penultimate anaesthetising pain block I was given before the transplant was an epidural. To insert the needle, I was told to arch my back like a cat. I have spent 95 per cent of my life co-habiting with felines and feel rather au fait with their behavioural habits; so, to be honest, I was not sure if they wanted me to stretch and flatten as if I was about to pounce and launch myself at the anaesthetist's gullet, stick one leg in the air and lick my own bum, or arch my back in fear as if a balloon had been burst within a 15-mile radius of where I lay. I went for the latter.

It all seemed like the end of a very long journey, and my

mind was awash with both dread and relief that an arduous chapter was coming to a close. I knew that the next 24 hours could both make or break me. I also knew that if this would be the last time I were ever to close my eyes, then perhaps – all things not said and not done – there were worse ways to go than under a general anaesthetic.

While such notions were of a greater distraction, it was quite genuinely the case that in another corner of my brain was the thought, *I'm glad I am going to be unconscious when they stick that tube up my willy.* Among the entire list of details I had to try and digest in the 45 minutes before being at the mercy of a scalpel-wielding surgeon, was that I'd have a catheter tube threaded down my urethra. There may have been some very important detail divulged to me during that prep talk, but my mind was totally distracted by that thought. It was a blessed relief when I discovered that I'd be fast asleep when that particular procedure was to take place.

By this stage in my life, I had not been for a wee for almost two years, and the idea that I might one day urinate again felt somewhat of a novelty. Only a few days after the operation, I was a catheter convert. Why isn't everyone attached to one all the time? You don't get the sensation of needing a wee, and you never get that 'busting' feeling. All you need to do is empty a bag of piss once in a while, or, as in my case, get a nurse to empty it for you – and piss bags can hold far more wee than a bladder. Bliss. I'm surprised they don't come as an optional extra with a La-Z-Boy recliner.

But the love affair with my catheter was short lived. As it turned out, it did have some logistical drawbacks. Despite feeling abso-bloody-lutely amazing, I was still quite happy to flomp on my bed and conserve energy to aid my convalescence. Nurses, however, wouldn't just leave me be: there was talk of bed sores and keeping airways open. The sooner I was up and about, the sooner I could be discharged. They often claimed that hospitals were the worst places for people recovering from trauma or surgery, something I couldn't really fathom at the time.

It took a team of four nurses and any visitors I had at my bedside who could be cajoled into assisting just to sit me up. Beyond my shredded stomach muscles was the issue of the tangle of cables, wires, and tubes, two of which (now giving me my bullet wound-looking scars) were always the responsibility of medical staff who handled them with extreme caution. Personally, I was more concerned with anyone wiggling my willy hose. If I ever find myself back in that situation, I hope by then that hospital beds will be wireless, and that I can be drip-fed via Bluetooth. Much of the sitting-up process involved choreographing the rolling of various machines and looping wires and tubes over the limbs and heads of the 'moving team'. I could have been a challenge in an escape room experience. It was a procedure done with exacting caution for the first two days before I was forced/bullied into moving to, not just an upright position in my bed, but also the previously unchartered territory of the nearby armchair.

＊＊＊＊＊

Despite all the praise and doorstep applauses NHS frontline nurses received in 2020, it is – I contest – only when you have been at the receiving end of their care that you realise quite what a unique breed they truly are. I myself am not cut out for a career which requires a uniform, they all seem a bit stress-y. So many necessitate a calm, comforting and caring demeanour when absolute blood-soaked hell is breaking loose, when life is at its most fragile and vulnerable. My role in life sometimes feels like it is to produce the 'blood-soaked hell', not deal with it.

How they undertake the tasks at hand with a cheery bedside manner, personally, I know my fight-or-flight instinct seems to have been replaced with a tears-and-tantrum knee-jerk reaction. I have met a number of tough-love matronly types over my years, and I've had a begrudging fondness for them all. There was one nurse in particular, Senior Sister Angela Green, who I would frequently see prior to my transplant, while I was on dialysis. She would always insist I came to routine appointments with an overnight bag, and upon her examination of my physical condition and blood test results – on a number of occasions at least – she would have to break it to me that the packing of that bag was not in vain. She knew how I hated that, but somehow she made it feel like she was admitting me to the ward because she, personally, actually cared. And how can you resent someone for that?

(I later found out, that before any family or friend came to visit me post-transplant, it was Angela who was the first to poke her nose around the high dependency ward's door to check up on me.)

And it was a nurse cut from the same cloth as Sister Angela Green who, having nagged me into submission, insisted I sat up in my bed and then make the arduous journey to the armchair. On the fourth day after the operation, just as she had propped me in the chair, she noticed a large, dark, wet patch around my pyjama crotch. She was with a trainee nurse, and between them, they detangled the mess of machine tubes from the catheter tube to discover the source of the leak.

'Oh!' exclaimed the matronly nurse, 'Does it normally look like that?' She was calm and measured, and I knew I had to tell her the truth. She was, without judgement, looking at my willy, which was a good three times its regular size, and not in an I've-got-a-matronly-nurse-wearing-latex-glove-fetish kind of way. Perhaps I should have given her a cheeky wink and replied, 'Yeah, and what of it?' But I think the apparent look of aghast shock on my face had already given the game away.

To make matters worse, and further impede any ruse that I could potentially brag about the size of my manhood, at that exact moment, an ex-girlfriend who happened to work as a nurse in another of the hospital's wards decided to pop her head around the curtain to see how I was getting on.

FOR THE (MEDICAL) RECORD

The bloodiest and body fluidiest end of my care was carried out by two hospitals in the UK; firstly, King's College Hospital in the south of London, where Professor Edmonds got me back on my wonky feet and where my kidney kaputness was first spotted, and secondly, Addenbrooke's Hospital in Cambridge. This is where my eyesight was saved, and my kidney needs in all their dialysing glory were taken over by the matronly Angela Green and her team. It was also where transplant surgeon Mr Gavin Pettigrew might well have been the person I told I had shit myself after I was roused from my anaesthetic-induced slumber. (I've always felt surgeons are cheated somewhat by their titles of Mr, Miss, Mrs, Ms rather than doctor, senior consultant, professor – all that hard work and training and they are effectively left with the same prefix as the person they are dissecting).

Both hospitals are in southeast England, and I lived pretty much halfway between them both. As the crow flies, King's College was 37 miles away, and Addenbrookes was 30. Fine on paper, or an Ordnance Survey map, or if you are a crow in flight, but it took over two hours door-to-door to get to King's, and about 45 minutes to get to Addenbrookes. The latter journey was an easy car jaunt for my mother or her partner, the former was a journey which, on occasion, involved hospital transport that took me on a veritable tour of the English countryside as it picked up other equally decrepit passengers – journeys often soundtracked by a mind-if-I smoke-mate taxi driver diatribe about 'broken Britain'. Alternatively, I could get a lift to my nearest railway station, limp on a train to London, a tube across the city, and another train to the hospital's general vicinity before a short walk to the front door. It was that journey which became more and more torturous the sicker and more infirm I became. On one occasion, when I was returning from a one-night stay for the purposes of a kidney biopsy, the train from London Liverpool Street to my town was full of commuters and there was standing room only. I leaned against the doors for support – it had only been a few hours since the procedure – with my overnight bag slung over my shoulders. It was stiflingly hot, and I was hemmed in so tight that any attempt to get to a disabled seat seemed futile, and I was not in the mood to explain why an apparently able-bodied thirty-something suddenly needed a seat. I could feel sweat trickle beneath my t-shirt. It was about 20 minutes later when I disembarked that I realised that it was not sweat, it was blood. A dark crimson blotch had stained my t-shirt, the top of my jeans and even dripped onto my orthopaedic sneakers.

But that was not the only drawback or the sole reason I requested all my care was transferred to Cambridge. The first time I was admitted to King's was when Professor Edmonds had noticed the glitch in my kidney function. I was still quite sprightly and not prone to lying in bed all day. It was hard to reconcile the fact that there could be something terminally wrong with me, bearing in mind the spring I had in my step – albeit a spring now cushioned by orthotics.

I was in a ward with at least ten other patients, and, as usual, I was the youngest by a country kilometre. While I think of myself as a chatty soul, in these situations, the company tends to be on the deaf side of the hearing spectrum. Not long after my afternoon arrival, a menu card was handed to me so I could choose my evening meal. I immediately ruled out the things I knew would make me puke, such as fish pie or anything which comes from an animal which I would wear the skin of on my feet, or the fleece of which I'd use to keep me snugly. That left a lot of options, none of which I recognised.

I challenge anyone to exorcise this sentiment from their psyche, but when you are at your most vulnerable, you want to be surrounded by the most familiar. The patients I shared the ward with reflected the community of the location of the hospital, and fittingly, the menu was curated around that community. Selecting a dish from a hospital menu didn't feel like the time to be adventurous. I know how this reads, and it is painful to admit, but I felt lonely. It was the first of many inpatient stays I had there, but the frustratingly long journey for my friends and family to visit and the isolation I felt became too much. One evening, I snuck out for a walk around the neighbouring city streets. It was the first time I had seen a 24-hour hair salon that could also transfer money to anywhere in the world. It was an area rich in a diversity I would otherwise embrace and explore, but now it just made me feel alone. After months of treatment at King's, both as a frequent in- and out-patient, it was clear I was seriously ill, and I needed to be on familiar territory if these were indeed to be my last days.

King's handed me over to Addenbrooke's after the dialysis line was finally secured into me, and I was fully trained (other than how to disconnect for a quick poo) on my dialysis machine. It was a relief for me, and also my mother, who had been running on fumes due to the endless schlepping to London to see me. Cambridge has always been my stomping ground of choice, and it is a city where I have many friends. The first time I had to be admitted to Addenbrooke's, I got chatting to a nurse who was making up a neighbouring bed. As it turned out, she had once shared a student home with the now wife of one of my oldest friends. Familiarity doesn't necessarily breed contempt, as it was turning out, Addenbrooke's is a huge employer, so it's no surprise that among its ranks I can include friends who work as porters, administrators, a psychotherapist, and a nurse – a nurse who had seen my willy for non-medical related reasons. When I had dated that very nurse, my willy had never, as far as I was aware, been the subject of so much concern, but now here we all were ...

*****

'Oh! Wow! Hi', my ex-girlfriend excitedly proclaimed. At first, I was mistaken into thinking she had joined the seemingly growing throng of people fixated on my urine-soaked groin, but as it turned out, she had recognised the trainee nurse who had recently been working on her ward. The whole sore and sordid affair was fast turning into an apparent social gathering, at which my willy-medical-emergency was not even the central talking point: the two nurses chatted away just metres from my inflated, red-sore willy and urine-soiled PJ bottoms.

After a fair amount of grappling and tube wiggling, the issue was resolved, but not without a small amount of willy-tissue grazing, abrasions and blood leakage. That all should be enough for any one willy to endure, but for mine, it was just the start of a very long and punishing journey.

During the last few days as a post-transplant inpatient, you are prepped for your Life 2.0. With the help of a physio, a dietician, and Pharmacy Girl, I was brought back to strength, educated on what not to eat (mainly grapefruit, from what I can recall) and loaded up on pills by the woman who apparently did not regard 'And I take these ones twice a day?' as the most flirty chat-up line she'd ever heard.

Within all that detail, the fact that I would have to return to hospital within a month or so to 'have the clip removed' was nonchalantly thrown into the mix. 'Clip? *What* clip?'. I had a few tubes and metal staples still holding me together, which I knew would be taken off and out as an outpatient, but I could see no clip.

What they don't tell you before you can back out of a life-saving double organ transplant, is that part of the overall procedure involves them using a plastic clip to help plumb the new kidney to your bladder. And once that plumbing is up and running, the clip can come out. Did I really have to go back under the knife so soon after having just been patched up after my last mauling?

'Oh, no', said the specialist, 'It is just a simple procedure where we nip in and get it out, it is not an operation'.

'Nip in and get it?' 'Nipping in and getting' are words usually reserved for buying a litre of milk from a corner shop, not retrieving a plastic paperclip from a bladder. The procedure was calmly explained to me, although receiving the detail filled me with an equal amount of terror as had the transplant surgery itself.

A tube is inserted up the urethra and a little grabby thing plucks the clip and drags it out. The whole thing would be livestreamed (more so the doctors could see what they were doing rather than for viewing pleasure). So, not only does a little grabby thing have to go 'up there', but also a *camera*?

'Nope, it's dark in there. We need to send a torch in as well.' Perhaps not a verbatim quote, but that was the gist. Why not send in a narrator as well and a guy holding a big fluffy microphone on a long boom handle? 'It's not as bad as childbirth', said the nurse some weeks after my initial discharge as she wheeled me towards the clip-removal procedure room, 'but it might feel that way when we pass the prostate gland', she added. The procedure went well, although it was noted that the injury caused by the catheter had not fully resolved itself, and there was some scarring and peripheral damage to the skin. Nothing urgent, nothing to worry about, and probably not a long-term problem. Yeah, sure, like I had never heard that before.

Just ten months later I was in a Swedish accident and emergency ward as a team of doctors and nurses stared at my willy, scratched their heads, and asked, with a collective wry smile, 'Did you do this on one of our women?'.

Since that initial trauma, my foreskin, which might never have been there if my supposed Jewish family tree ran down the right branch, was now an immovable object. Ever since I was a teenager I've been grappling with my willy in the interests of pleasure and 'I-wonder-if-it-can' during experimental moments of my formative years. Since the initial swelling had gone down and the abrasions healed, I really had done everything I could think of to get it to cooperate, but my foreskin just wouldn't budge.

I doubt I could've gotten this on prescription, but as it turned out, sex was the answer. Having jetted off to Sweden for the first time, full of expectations for this blossoming relationship, within a day of arrival, the issue was resolved. Sort of. The skin had effectively folded in on itself. It wasn't painful, but now it was stuck again – at the other end, and at the base of, my willy. Hours after the 'resolving incident', it did appear that more blood was flowing in than was flowing out – my foreskin was acting like a makeshift cock ring. In the end, we called for medical help and were surprised by the urgency in the voice of the person who'd picked up our call. We went straight to casualty, where the awaiting team of medics pondered on who or what I 'broke' it on.

It took about 30 minutes, a copious amount of opiate-based painkillers, and a lot of 'nearly theres' before the team did the least erotic imaginable 'tug' to get everything back to where it should be. We had a good laugh about it in the taxi home, but that was probably more a result of the drugs and relief than anything else. The doctors advised me that a medical circumcision was definitely the best course of action. Upon my return to the UK, I visited my GP who agreed with the Swede's consensus.

My circumcision was now in the laps of the Waiting List Gods, but obviously this was something I wanted sorted urgently, as that episode was most definitely not an experience I wanted to repeat. However, on the first night of my second visit to Sweden, the exact thing happened again. At least this time we knew what to do, and back to the emergency ward we went. The fact that it was a different team of doctors and nurses was a minor saving grace.

A date for the circumcision was finally set. I kept the whole operation pretty much on the down-low, not through any sense of shame or embarrassment but rather due to the fact that my family and friends had already had to endure so much stress with my medical mishaps that I'd rather just minimise any more oh-god-he's-back-in-hospital-again provoked sleepless nights.

To ensure an easy in-and-out day procedure, I opted for a local anaesthetic (a general would've required an overnight stay) – a decision the doctor questioned with a raised eyebrow. The procedure itself took around 45 minutes, and while I was entirely conscious, the local anaesthetic meant all I could really feel was the elbow of the surgeon as he rested himself on my inner thigh. I had been wheeled into a room which appeared as an unnecessarily large operating theatre. However, at one point, another doctor popped his head around the door to inquire as to the whereabouts of a colleague. The surgeon, my willy in hand, gestured with a 'reverse nod' that the colleague being asked after was in an adjoining room, and it was okay to use the fire escape door at the other end of the room to get to her. At this point, the doctor walked past me, apologised for the intrusion, witnessed the business end of what was occurring, and did the kind of quick step you do to indicate you are making at least a quasi-effort to hurry yourself along.

It was The Willy Experience which dovetailed my final NHS procedure and my first venture into the Swedish healthcare system. I have so much to thank both systems for. Obviously, it is the NHS who should take the lion's share of the gratitude, but I have encountered many amazing doctors and specialists along the way, on both sides of the North Sea.

Whether you are a clapper or a complainer, it is hard to deny that both countries have fantastically advanced welfare states and healthcare systems. If you don't agree, and you live in the Global North, then open your eyes. You probably have better sight than I do – use it. Since gaining dual citizenship, it has always felt such a privilege to be the holder of two passports for two countries where I know I will be so well looked after.

I have trusted them with my life and my willy, and they have not failed me. I am happy to entrust my body into their hands to do as they will in a bid to keep me alive for as long as possible. I sometimes feel like I've already donated my body to medical research, what with all the doctors' fingers I've had shoved up and down various orifices. If I ever got any tattoos, I might consider a number of 'exit only' guidelines scattered around my battered body. With all that has happened to me comes an unwavering level of trust: I will do what they tell me to do, and I will un-flinchingly follow their lead. No matter how counterintuitive their actions may seem, I understand that they are for my best, that those actions are carried out with a wealth of knowledge and experience behind them.

And that's the way I have always felt, until …

The pivotal moment was December 16, 2020, when the crest of Sweden's second wave was at tsunami proportions. It was at the time that hospital staff were nudged into wearing a face mask if they were within a two-metre radius of a patient.

On this day of reckoning, I had two early morning appointments. The first was with my orthotics specialist who had agreed I could have some new winter walking boots made. I am not really the walking boot type, but so much of my social present and future was spent outside and, in addition, my wife has a penchant for foraging in forests and on occasion drags me along if she finds a suitably disabled-friendly woodland path.

You would have thought that any profession which requires the working day to be spent at the business end of diseased feet would, by default, warrant a face mask, but today was the first day I ever saw my specialist wearing one, and on this occasion, her trainee as well. In fact, not only masks, judging by their attire you'd have guessed they thought I had taken a Novichok foot bath before my appointment – masks, visors, gloves, aprons, the whole kit and caboodle.

So I was in a mask, and they were PPE'd to the hilt. The bits I use to breathe in airborne viruses were at one end of my body, and the bits the specialists were interested in were at the other end. Everything felt safe enough.

The next appointment was to get my monthly blood test. I was a bit early, so I cycled a lap around the hospital grounds to ensure the minimal amount of time was spent loitering in a waiting room where, by its very nature, I'd only be sharing air with people suffering varying degrees of disease and degradation, and staff who come into daily contact with such unfortunate souls.

When it finally came to my turn, I was led to a private room where a young Swedish woman with a tightly tied ponytail prepped the vials and asked me the routine questions: Had I fasted? When did I take my last tablets?

She had spiked my arm and was just attaching the first vial – one of seven – when she turned away and expelled a light cough. Not a phlegmy hack, but a cough all the same. Such a cough, even in an outdoor social situation, was now to be frowned upon, never mind in a medical setting. She apologised and then continued. Moments later, she coughed again, this time both turning away and coughing into the crease of her elbow.

I asked whether she was okay, and she insisted she was fine, proffering as a reason for her cough a reaction to wearing a face mask for such a long period of time. Now, I can totally sympathise with intensive care staff who have to wear full-on PPE for 23-hour shifts, but she was wearing a regular medical paper-y mask, and it had, after all, only just gone 9am.

She once again insisted she was fine and continued the blood-letting before finally succumbing to such a coughing fit that she required a glass of water. At this point, I am quite literally flabbergasted, and I don't mind admitting it, scared, upset, and annoyed. She tucked the mask under her chin (one of the greater face mask faux pas, as we are now all aware), had a slurp of water, pulled the mask back up, alcohol gelled her hands, and returned to the task at hand.

And then started coughing again. I had already asked her if she was okay, so instead I decided to tell her, 'You're not okay'. She caught the attention of a colleague and asked her to take over. She left. I was bereft.

I had felt so privileged to live in a country where my routine appointments and the monitoring of my various conditions were being upheld during a time when so many of the healthcare services were being squeezed. I am not saying that neither the NHS nor the Swedish healthcare authorities are without their critics, and, objectively, I know they are both woefully under-funded, but from my perspective, I only exist because they do.

I have never, ever questioned a medically qualified opinion, never veered away from guidance given by someone wearing a white lab coat, nurses uniform or scrubs. I've felt scared before – and never so much as when a surgeon carved away at my willy while nonchalantly chatting to his colleague – but I never, ever regarded a paid-up member of staff as a threat, until now.

Maybe that nurse delegated the job because she could see the fear in my eyes, but I am fairly sure that I saw her leaving early for the day after my blood was letted. Was I the last patient she saw before she was signed off sick? I'll never know. Only time would tell what harm she may have caused.

Chapter 10
Have yourself a Covid-y little Christmas

I could say that my total apathy towards Christmas is down to diminishing marginal returns of utility, or to put it more succinctly, being a grownup. Perhaps it is the fact that Tess and I have opted for a child-free family unit, meaning we are not culturally bound to feign a belief in Santa, pointlessly relocate an elf every bloody morning before 'poppet' wakes up, or fret that our kid's nativity play is going to end up on the darknet for a waiting ring of paedos with a penchant for seven-year-old shepherds. It might be that we are both ardent atheists and anti-consumerists, but I think, in all honesty, we just can't be bothered with it all. Even people who try to 'escape Christmas' with a far-flung holiday to a Muslim or Hindu country seem to spend more time and energy on avoiding Christmas than many do on actual, well, Christmas.

However, what Tess and I can be bothered about are our families. Both of us have one sibling, both our respective siblings are older brothers, and both our older brothers have children. My older brother has a wife, while Tess's older brother is a serial monogamist and is seemingly always in the embryonic throes of a relatively fresh relationship around the festive period. My brother's in-laws celebrate a more traditional, albeit Catholic-flavoured, Christmas, with both late night and early morning church services, later topped off with some by proxy cardinal sinning via the medium of an EastEnders season special. And it is this side of his family where my brother and his brood choose to spend every Christmas. Two days later they descend upon my mother's place for Christmas 2.0.

It is hit and miss whether Tess's brother will show up at their parents', but invariably, it is a miss. Tess and I, therefore, independently make the choice to spend that time of year with our respective elders. We know our siblings will either be a no-show or a tokenistic pop-in. 2020 was to be our tenth Christmas as a couple, and up until 2020, we had spent precisely zero of those Christmases together. It is a quirk of our relationship, perhaps borne out of both nonchalance and an egotistical notion that Tess's parents want to spend this time with her, and my mother and her partner want to spend the time with me. An assumption that does actually pan out in reality.

I tend to view my trip back as just another excuse to catch up with my friends and family. All I want to do is wrap myself in a cloak of apathy and make the time as similar as possible as any other trip back to the UK. Christmas, however, never fails to frustrate, as it wheedles its way into my routines with reduced rail services and close friends absent because they are spending this Christmas with 'his side of the family in the Cotswolds'.

But there is more to it than that. While I hate my brain for thinking like this, my brain has a mind of its own, and for every obligatory card bought and sent, every gift purchased and received, an imaginary profit and loss account sheet is drafted. And once the tinsel is torn down, after every Christmas that ledger in my mind seems to end with a financial report detailing a net fiscal loss.

Within the realms of privilege lies a spectrum of financial security. Not for one nanosecond would I lay claim to having experienced anything close to abject poverty. But relative poverty? Well, that's another matter, and it is a matter which supersedes poor career choices and misfortune – living with disease and disability are not known money-spinners. Not many get-rich-quick bestsellers suggest multiple organ failure as a fast-track to success, and no one has ever gone into the Dragon's Den and asked for half a million quid for a 50 per cent share of their liver.

In all honesty, the profit and loss account was probably first set up when I was a clichéd, poverty-stricken student. If my brother wanted a new thermos flask for Christmas, then would I have enough money left in my coffers to buy Aaron T. Beck's *Cognitive Therapy and the Emotional Disorders* book, which was a required text for the upcoming semester? I wasn't the only one affected. I remember a nursing student sobbing in my room after receiving a pair of fluffy slippers from her father despite having asked for money to buy course literature. 'I can't even wear them, they look like vaginas', she blubbered. Christmas: misplaced spending on such an epic and, practically, global scale.

Years later, and after the disease-enforced demise of my career, no one really expected much from me as I survived hand-to-mouth on benefits and benefactors, but I'd still somehow run at a loss. The financial elements of Christmas, however, paled into insignificance once the sickness's stranglehold tightened. The first botched attempt to insert a peritoneal dialysis tube into my lower abdomen took place late December 2007. The Christmas 'holiday season' that year consisted of an appointment on December 22nd, December 24th, December 31st, January 4th, and January 5th. All those appointments were at the tail end of the arduous slog to the hospital in the south of London and required battling a severely depleted train service and exorbitantly priced London black cabs at a time of the year when all drivers had set their rates to, from what I could tell, 'fleece the crap out of the passenger'. At the time, I was suffering from acute motion sickness, and while I know this will read as gross exaggeration, I can assure you that, if anything, this is an underestimate: I'd probably dry heave about every ten seconds, and that did not tail off, no matter the length of the journey. I'd take a plastic carrier bag with me whenever I got in a car, although lumpy, wet bits were rarely regurgitated, it was more of an insurance and a way to reassure the driver I wasn't going to soil their floor mats. You can imagine how the average London cabbie regards a perma-puking passenger.

It was a time of not only the inherent physical painful symptoms of hitherto healthy organs but also a time of deep psychological trauma as I was fitted with a disfiguring plastic tube poking out of my abdomen. Not knowing when, or indeed if, that tube would ever be removed weighs heavy on the mind. But to everyone else in my social circles, other than the very closest to me, 2007 was just another Christmas.

The following Christmas, when the at-first horrific realities of a life of connecting to a dialysis machine every night were now just as routine as most would consider popping an Alka-Seltzer as a pre-emptive strike against a possible office party-induced hangover, a whole new host of horrors awaited. It'd be unfair to suggest that any effort made by my mother was nothing but tokenistic, but when a close family member is sat at the dining table looking as pale as a slice of turkey meat, it must be hard to muster up much enthusiasm, particularly when most of the traditional Christmas culinary fare lay way beyond my dialysis dietary restrictions. Even the simplest of seasonal pleasures was stripped away from me. A rule-breaking morsel of turkey and a few roast spuds – that was pretty much it for me. Eating the dried fruit in a mince pie or Christmas pudding – going by the dialysis cookbooks the hospital gave me – would have been as fatally akin to me seasoning my meal with strychnine.

In addition, my mother could not drink because I had to be back home long before midnight in fear that, unlike Cinderella, who would be returned to her normal, healthy, albeit sad self, I'd be turned into, after a while at least, a corpse. Sleeping for a hundred years might be a wistful trope in a fairy tale, but in my reality, it was a coma. I only ever had one Christmas when I was actually on dialysis, but it's a Christmas I remember more than any other. That was in 2008. By 2009 I had met Tess, but it was only in 2020 that, for the first time, we were forbidden by both governments and, indeed, by our own virus-fearing parents, to spend the occasion at their respective homes. Tess is just a short car journey from her folks, exacerbating her frustration with a so-near-yet-so-far element. My trip back to the UK always presented a stubborn hurdle – or 'Denmark', as it is known by most, which I had to jump, seeing as the most efficient route for my trips to the UK are via Copenhagen. In 2020 it was more of a pole vault than a hurdle, as Denmark, along with much of the EU, was rightfully aghast at the spiking cases in the UK. It was battening down its hatches, so even if I had managed to get back to the UK, there was every chance I'd not be able to get back to Sweden in the unforeseeable future.

So, seeing as everything else in the year had been turned on its head, I decided to enter this season of good tidings with an upbeat, and partially forced, sense of joy. Tess and I would make a go of it. We had bought a two-metre tree, which was tastefully decorated by Tess's artistic eye, and made sure our online food order was placed in good time to ensure all the Swedish traditional trimmings were locked and loaded in our larder.

On any other year, I'd have flown to the UK a week before Christmas to guarantee I could catch up with anyone who was planning to spend their Christmas away from our traditional stomping ground. That socialising window is, traditionally, my favourite time of the season. Unfortunately, not only was that denied by travel restrictions, but also work had been nothing but a total bastard, and it was only on December 23rd that I had achieved the Herculean feat of okaying my out-of-office autoreply. The day had been spent preparing a report for my manager and overly prepping for the first weeks of January to ensure as smooth a start as possible when back 'in the office' – an office in our flat that I could now turn back into a cosy room which is at its most enjoyable when I am snuggled up on an armchair in front of a faux-flaming heater and reading a good book on my e-reader (which affords me the luxury of enlarging the text to a size my piss-poor eyes are comfortable with).

Being the good Lutherans the Swedes once were, the jovialities of a feast, crap telly, a board game and too much commercially produced moonshine (or snaps, as the Swedes call it these days) are held on Christmas Eve, with Christmas Day itself having more of a, for my ethnocentric British brain at least, Boxing Day kind of vibe. The 23rd therefore, feels very much like the 24th in the UK.

At about 3.30pm, as I sat in shallow thought and gazed at a recently shut down blank screen, the strong smell of frying onions wafted in from the kitchen. Tess was preparing the 'julbord' ('jul' = Christmas, 'bord' = table, 'julbord' = what the Swedes eat instead of roast turkey and all the trimmings) for the following day's feast. I was hardly lost in a moment of profound contemplation of 2020, rather more of a 'thank fuck I've got two weeks off work'; either way, the moment was broken by the shuffling of Tess's slippers as she hesitantly and sheepishly crept to the threshold of the room. She delivered a muted, attention-seeking cough and, with a look of 'I've just broken that family heirloom your dad gave you on his death bed', said, 'I can't smell the onions'.

She. Could. Not. Smell. The. Onions. I could smell the onions, judging by the cat's twitching nose, he could smell the onions. I imagine Will and Brandy, the neighbours across the hall, could smell the onions, but Tess? Tess could not smell the onions. This was it: had we been breached? Had Covid miraculously wormed its way into our home?

The mood went from 'winding down' to 'wound up to the point of breaking'. She felt fine, she claimed at least, and insisted her temperature of 37.5c was normal for her ('That's why I always feel cold', she proffered for mitigating circumstances – a barbed reminder of all the times I've questioned why she would wear 'that' coat in 'this' heat).

But we both knew it; this was among the first of the now notorious nasal symptoms of The Second Biggest C killer.

Frustration, fear, anger, panic, divorce, burn at the stake? What to feel and what to do were soon joined by 'how?'. *How* – after treating every foreign object like it was weapon-grade uranium and everyone who was not a 'me' or a 'Tess' as a 100% guaranteed source of our, or at least my, doom – *could this have happened*?

The how, however, then became an afterthought. The real issue here was, did I have it, and if not, how could I avoid contracting it? What else could I have done? We were living in a practically hermetically sealed living space with a decontamination porch area entrance that had such a strict protocol it could be the blueprint for a Hospital of Tropical Diseases' We-Don't-Know-What-These-People-Have-or-Why-They-are-Turning-Purple-and-Then-Exploding pop-up ward.

Further measures were implemented: separate beds and sleeping quarters, separate towels, making sure you definitely took the right toothbrush out of the mug, me giving shifty back-the-fuck-off glares if she came within my own personal space, a personal space considerably more spacious than the UK government's guidelines of two metres. So, this was to be our first Christmas 'together'?! Well, we were hoping it was going to be special ...

Tess continued to feel fine all evening, although increasingly preoccupied by her loss of smell, sniffing every morsal she ate and proclaiming again and again, 'Nope, still nothing', then going into the kitchen and opening various jars and boxes with growing frustration and a moan of 'Oh no! Not even coffee!'.

On 24th December, Sweden's 'Christmas Day', we both

woke up with our best brave faces on and decided to push through with whatever the day was to throw at us. If disease-spreading damage was to be done, we were probably too late to stop it. Even so, the only damage we were really considering was me getting Covid. Nothing else.

Tess, in a festive yet futile attempt to bring some seasonal joy, plugged in the Christmas tree lights. I heard a yelp, a few crashes, bangs, the sound of rolling baubles on floorboards, and a multilingual tirade of expletives. She had been thrown across the room by an electric shock from the lights, which had not been used for more than 20 years. The day went downhill from there.

Despite our, but mainly my, utter nonchalance for the day, we continued to soldier on and participated in some of the Scandi traditions. The Swedes, as far as I can tell, celebrate all their major holidays with exactly the same culinary bland core of pickled herring and potatoes – foods my father would sentimentalise while my brother and I recoiled in horror as he recalled childhood memories of World War Two and living off food rations. Fortunately, Tess is an accomplished cook and had curated from the array of foods served up on the average julbord, a suitably presentable Adrian-friendly feast. Every mouthful I had, while being delicious, was laced with a fear that my lunch companion might be infecting me while I dined; she hadn't been wearing latex gloves while she sliced and diced the ingredients. Meanwhile, Tess sat glumly staring at her plate while giving a frustrated huff every time she failed to taste her smoked salmon.

After lunch, the Swedes retire to watch an hour of Donald Duck cartoons and clips of old Walt Disney classics, the same cartoons and clips year in and year out. The show has remained largely unchanged since its inception in 1958. I'd say that is beyond peculiar, but then I guess in the UK, loyal subjects sit around watching the Queen prattle on about the year just gone; although at least in the UK you can try and guess which one of her family has pissed her off the most by figuring out who is absent from the family photos on an in-shot occasional table or ponder on whether Prince Harry ever fired up Pornhub on his gold-plated Apple Mac and had a "browse" while perched on 'Nanny's special Christmas chair'. It occurred to me that it didn't really matter whether I was in the UK or Sweden, the day is almost custom made to frustrate me, whether I was distracted by debt-fuelled depression, on dialysis, or watching Donald Duck.

*****

Everyone loves to play boardgames around Christmas, and this year we decided to plump for a bespokely updated version of that age old classic, Cluedo. Only we called it Co-vido. In this version, we were the victims, and the aim was to discover which one of our dastardly friends had dunnit/speadit. The game descended into us admonishing each other's 'reckless' actions which could, potentially, lead to our mutual dooms.

Retracing our steps from the week before Christmas revealed, however, that I was the only one who had actually been in contact with anyone in a non-digital form. Could it be, that I unknowingly already had it? Covid, just like the dad of the chap's birthday we were 'celebrating', certainly does seem to move in mysterious ways. We unscrupulously assessed when and with whom I might have fallen foul of.

Suspect: Daniel

Location: A well-ventilated function room

Weapon: A takeaway falafel

Just over a week before Christmas, I had been to an impromptu, intimate Christmas soiree (mates drinking) with two close colleagues-cum-friends. Daniel had chosen one of our workplace's large function rooms as a suitable meeting point. The room has ridiculously high ceilings and a kitchen area we could use to prepare the hors d'oeuvre (individual bowls of crisps). I had arrived late and upon joining the others, a bottle of wine and a bottle of hand gel were, in tandem, shunted towards me, thus enabling a sanitised pour. Moments later, a takeaway falafel was drawn to my attention. Was this our downfall? Ingredients bought by a stranger, prepared by a stranger, and wrapped and bagged by a stranger – was Daniel the unwitting conduit between me and a coughing, spluttering fast food employee? Possibly. I nuked the falafel to the point of inedibility in the microwave to be on the safe side. I don't think it could've been Daniel. Next!

Suspect: Janni

Location: A park bench

Weapon: Something to keep our bums dry

A few days after the falafel, I had met with my friend Janni for a coffee. We opted to rendezvous in the fresh air of the park which runs between our two apartment blocks. We both entered a café to buy takeaway drinks and were the only ones in there, in situ for only a matter of moments. Janni, myself and the woman behind the counter, all maintained more than the recommended dose of distance.

However, upon leaving – and having decided on a wet park bench as our resting spot – Janni produced from her bag two plastic foam seat cushions which we could use to keep our bums dry.

Weren't toilet seats thought to be partially to blame for the spread of the HIV virus back in the 80s? Could waterproof bum protectors be the new scaremongering conspiracy theory? What if this virus could be spread by sharing a bum cushion? I didn't need to fall back on my rudimentary science education to rule out this ludicrous notion. Besides, Janni's partner is also a bit of a high risker, so she probably keeps her bum-protecting seat cushions in a suitably sanitised bum cushion container. It definitely was not Janni.

Suspect: Maja

Location: A café's outdoor seating area

Weapon: A book about the Roma community in the city of Malmö

Maja is the Swedish teacher who I see every other week. I had started my online lessons with her during the first wave, but we had been meeting in the flesh since that wave had receded and the coast was looking clear. She is more than aware of my predicament and is the first person to cancel a lesson if one of her brood comes back from school with even a whiff of a sniffle. She always goes into the café to buy the coffee to ensure I don't have to take that risk and uses alcohol gel before ferrying my latte from the counter to our table.

However, on this occasion she presented me with a book which she herself had written. The book was a series of conversations with local Roma people, which made the individuals relatable to the wider community and beyond.

She lent me the book in the hope it might inspire me to write my own book (this book), with the ulterior motive that I might also learn from the Swedish text. I guess corona could be transported by paperback, but my hectic schedule at that point meant the book sat in my bag for two days before I had a chance to flick through it. There is no way the virus could have survived that long, even if it had laced the pages in the first place. It wasn't Maja.

Suspect: Patrick

Location: A rickety table on a cobbled street

Weapon: A disappointingly small and over-priced latte

Just a few days before Christmas, I had met with my friend Patrick. He has all the makings of a super-spreading supremo and is not even in the shadow of a risk group. He is the owner of two (more often than not) snotty young boys and is, seemingly, always up for a mingle – ongoing plague or not. Indeed, on this occasion, arranged in order for me to buy him a belated birthday brunch, he looked every inch the post-Brit Awards Noel Gallagher, sporting aviator sunglasses despite the overcast skies of the day. He was done with his office job for the year and was diving headfirst into the festive spirit. During the course of our socially distanced breakfast, he recounted a litany of crimes against the pandemic that he had committed; not boasting, I should clarify but rather simply regaling. He was, as we conversed, hungover from an indoor drinking session with his neighbour which, judging by the frazzled look of him, had only come to a conclusion hours before we met. With all that in mind, he was always insistent on being hyper careful when in my presence. Despite the odds, it was not last night's booze I could smell on him but rather the remnants of the over-zealously applied alcohol gel that he had slathered himself in just to bring me my frothy coffee. It, probably, was not Patrick.

Suspect: Johanna

Location: The pavement outside our flat

Weapon: A bottle of moonshine

The last person I had seen before we battened down the Christmas hatches (and before we knew we were potentially battening in the virus with us), was Johanna. Johanna is a friendly colleague and a congenial friend, and true to those traits, she had messaged me to tell me she was cycling over to present me with a gift. Johanna is, from all I know of her, a highly gregarious soul, but reckless and feckless? I can't see it. She had concocted some homemade glögg (Sweden's version of mulled wine) and presented it to me with a heads-up warning as to its lethality. I, in turn, had given her a bag of recently foraged and dried mushrooms. The transaction was carried out with all exacting attention to detail one would have witnessed during a Cold War spy exchange. It felt safe. Besides, there is no way Tess could be presenting symptoms one day later had it been Johanna who was the infecting host.

Our game was played sporadically throughout the day, everyone was assessed – the incriminations flowed and flowed.

I wasn't really expecting a 60-year-old Donald Duck cartoon to distract us, or even our mood-lightening attempt to find the culprit who had infected at least one of us. Everything was laced with an anxiety that I could be spending the upcoming New Year's Eve consuming my oxygen from a ventilator rather than the bubbles in a Champagne flute. I was quite genuinely terrified by this prospect now I knew there was a very high chance the infection was running amok in our flat. There was also a sense of complacency that there was very little we could do about it if it was.

*****

Beyond the stress that Tess might be in the process of killing her husband, was the sense of displacement she had felt for spending the first Christmas in her life away from her parents. But today was my turn, it was now December 25th – UK Christmas Day.

Tess continued to protest she was still feeling entirely fine, although her temperature was now running at 37.8c – a number given, certainly by the NHS in the UK, as a bit of a red alert. I had not stopped my daily cycles, but now there were two health benefits from such exercise: aerobic and keeping away from my wife. My mind often meanders as I zip and zoom along the city's cycle paths, and that day was no different.

FOR THE (MEDICAL) RECORD

How many times had I been asked if I was feeling any symptoms over the last year? Certainly every time I had gone for a blood test or a foot appointment. And how many times had I lied and said, 'No'? The reality is that – certainly in the winter months – I am almost always a bit snotty. I am not coughing, I am not sneezing, I don't have a temperature, I am just a bit bunged-up or runny-nosed. Whether this is caused by cold air tickling my nasal snot glands or whether it is just a hyper mild infection, I never really know. I genuinely don't pay such symptoms any attention. It is part of my course – my every wintery day lived experience – so I really don't feel like I am properly lying when I say, 'no'.

Every two or three years I might get a bad cold. They feel like they come on in a matter of moments and when they hit, they hit hard. The last time it happened was on New Year's Eve 2018. Tess had sent me on a mad morning dash for a shopping run to buy some forgotten ingredients for our ritual slap-up dinner for two. As I left the store I could sense a feeling of not-quite-rightness; a minute later as I unlocked my bike, I knew I was coming down with something. It was a ten-minute cycle home and with every push of the pedal I could feel my body weakening, the energy sapping, the infection gathering strength and pace. I made it home, threw the food onto the kitchen table, declared I needed to lie down and slept until Tess, about eight hours later and wearing her poshest eating-in clothes, prodded me awake in the hope I could at least join her for the dinner she had spent all day slaving over. I made it to the table, ate what I could and was in bed long before the midnight hour. And I stayed in bed for a week, not a five-day working week, a full-on seven-day calendar week. I got up only to force down the sustenance I knew my body needed to recover, and then up again for the bodily functions I needed to rid myself of the bits of sustenance my body felt were surplus to regaining full health requirements. If my blood temperature reaches 39.8c for two days or more, I am under strict instructions to contact my specialist transplant consultant, but if my blood temperature reaches 39.8c, I don't have the strength to pick up a phone – Tess would have to take over. Fortunately, it has never come to that, but this is what a bad cold is like for me. Not flu, a cold, just a bad cold. It takes an additional week for me to build up enough strength to leave the house. If I feel even the slightest hint that I am coming down with something, I slam on the brakes, go straight to bed, take two paracetamols, and let whatever immune system I have left do whatever it can – nine times out of ten that works. One time out of ten, it doesn't.

So day-to-day winter snot comes and day-to-day winter snot goes, as long as it is not accompanied by that inkling of dread that it could sneak though my immune system do I start to fret. But snot is not binary, it is a spectrum. So, on a 1 to 10 scale, 1 is the type of snot I get when I cycle for more than five minutes in the winter. Level 10 is death bed snot, and when it spikes at Level 10, snot is the least of my problems. In fact, the higher up the Snot Spectrum I go, the less snot there actually is. I'd say if it reaches 4, I do the paracetamol and early night procedure. Levels 2 to 3 are just 'blah whatever' snot.

As I cycled on that Christmas Day afternoon and built up some Level 1 snot along the way, my mind traced back to any chink in our alcohol-gelled armour as to how either one of us could have gotten infected. Then it occurred to me, the weekend before Christmas (Christmas day was on a Friday, that year), my snot levels were running at around Level 3.5, as too, were Tess's (not that she measures her snot in levels, but we had both acknowledged something was askew). Either way, it was a short-lived snot spike, by Monday they were back to their normal 0-1 levels. But that weekend was three days after the blood test with The Coughing Nurse. Had I cracked it? From the off, there was much talk of Covid's biphasic nature; many spoke of suffering a mild infection, seemingly recovering and then,

wallop, you were in intensive care saying your final fare-
wells to your friends and family via the medium of face-
time technology.

It was the best theory we had so far. If this theory was
correct, then Tess would be in her second phase, and I was,
well – *well*. Good for me. But alas, the theory was almost
immediately debunked. As I cycled home that Christmas
Day, snot levels went from 1.1 to 2.7. Then to Level 4. In
about twenty minutes.

Was this it? Whatever it was, we both now had it. We
had been trying to arrange a Covid test for Tess since the
first symptoms had nestled in, but all The Ables who were
hellbent on selfishly saving their Christmases had soaked
up any available testing time slots, ruling out any such
peace of mind/I-should-probably-get-my-last-will-and-
testament-in-order test results for us.

I could not *not* call my Mum on UK Christmas Day, so I
made a point of doing so before Level 4 increased to feverish numbers. I could feel my muscles aching as I held the
phone on video-call mode at an angle which allowed Tess
and myself to both fit in the screen. The minute I closed
the chat, content that I had duped my mother into thinking that all was well, I went to bed.

*****

Well, this is new. I had woken hours later with symptoms
which overlapped but were not entirely consistent with
neither cold or flu nor Covid. Sure, I had a high temperature and aches, but the pain seemed to penetrate from my
pasty outer shell to my re-wired and weakened very central core. My skin was on fire, and so sensitive that even

putting on a t-shirt caused a discomfort, which felt like an ISIS and/or CIA torture technique. What really crippled, or crippled me even further, was the excruciating pain in my bones: the pain jabbed and sneaked up on me without warning or a run-up. I was in agony. However, my sense of smell was intact, and there was no trace of a cough. Meanwhile Tess, just two days after failing to whiff the overwhelming aroma of frying onions, now had a healthy body temperature and was feeling absolutely fine.

I took the requisite dose of paracetamol and went to bed, hoping the tried and tested would be the treatment required. The following day my temperature had subsided and symptoms had started to fade, albeit my skin was still ablaze if it came into contact with anything but, well, air. Tess – who was still smelling everything like an over-excited puppy – hesitantly cried out, 'I think I got a whiff of garlic!'.

What was this? Neither of us had had a cough, neither of us really had any of the main suspect symptoms other than Tess's loss of smell. We double-downed on finding a place to get tested and eventually booked ourselves in for the following day, December 27th.

I can't say I was not so worried that I didn't have all my various specialist consultants' contact details to hand on my bedside table, laying among the detritus of popped paracetamol packages, but the skin pain was quickly becoming manageable. By the time we got to the drive-thru test centre, we had pretty much concluded that whatever it was, it was not Covid. Two days later, now on December 29th, Tess hurriedly cranked open her laptop after receiving a text from the health authorities alerting her that she had received her result. One gasp of astonishment and a 'fuuuucking hell' later, the result was revealed: POSITIVE. I raced to open my inbox, and there was my result: POSI-TIVE. We had it or had had it, although we really had no idea where we were on the corona timeline.

It almost felt surreal, all the paranoid alcohol gelling, the Fort Knox-esque protocol for entering our home, all the double-the-distance distancing, me holding my breath every time I walked or cycled past anyone, the bastard-cold meetups with friends outside cafes in the bleak mid-Swed-ish winter. And to avoid what? A few days of discomfort? Only during one of those days did I consider myself not perky enough for my daily dose of cycling. Sure, I might have felt at the time the pain was 'excruciating', but what-ever it was, it was short-lived, and in retrospect, when you have felt the levels of pain that I have felt, 'excruciating' is not actually that bad – you know you are in real pain when you just want the offending body part to be amputated/removed or, even more drastically, consider lopping it off/digging it out yourself. Of course I was braced for any sniff of another symptom, but it, or they, never came. And then the dawning realisation: in a weird way, Tess and I felt cheated. Weren't we supposed to have suffered more? All that time and money spent on not getting ill, and when we finally got it, with the benefit of hindsight, it amounted to a minor blip which, by happy coincidence, did not eat into the time we had reserved for anything more than sitting around on our arses and eating anyway.

So, how wrong we were with our skew on the boardgame Cluedo, in fact, this could now read as more of an Agatha Christie Christmas Special plot twist: those who were try-ing to expose the suspects were … dun-dun-duuuun … the very ones who were the culprits. Perhaps the greatest twist, and certainly a rather mundane one at that, is that the 'victims' were fine, and the culprits were found to have committed no crimes. No deaths, no arrests, no charges. Nothing to see here. I had contacted all the one-time suspects – all were doing just fine.

*****

(Weeks later, my consultant requested I had an antibody test, it was then confirmed – seeing as my blood was writhing with them — I had indeed both contracted and recovered from SARS-CoV-2.)

Chapter 11
Help

Toby: I dunno, probably around 7

Me: And I can definitely get a lift home?

Toby: Yeah, either Liam or me can drop you back

It was May 14th, 2009, and I was texting one of my closest pals, Toby. I've known Toby since 1997, when he sloped into a charity bookstore I was 'managing'. He was back home for summer, in the midst of his degree, and his mother had asked him to get out from under her feet and find a job. I told him we only had volunteer positions; he started the next day. Since then, well, I can't say we've become as thick as thieves, because neither of us are that thick, and we are both relatively law-abiding; neither are we blood brothers, because neither of us are big on blood-letting, despite the number of times I've had my blood drawn. We're just very, very good friends. If I had to design a perfect friend, it'd walk, talk, and do like Toby. His then fiancée, and now wife, Aine, had not long before this text exchange took place, offered me one of her kidneys. The pair of them were a huge support during my darkest days.

We often communicated with a flurry of text messages, sometimes we gave a running commentary on X-Factor contestants as we watched Saturday night telly in our respective homes, but on this occasion, it was to clarify the logistical necessities to get me – at the apex of my ill health – to a quiz night that was taking place in a community centre the coming Saturday. It was a Thursday evening, around 8.30pm, and I was sitting on my living room floor, perched up against an armchair trying to navigate my body as close as possible to the gas heater. I was always cold. Always being cold was either a symptom of my organ failure or a side effect of one or all the medications I was on. I can't remember which, I just remember always being cold. So cold, in fact, that I had qualified for a benefit to aid with my heating bill – I was local government registered 'cold'. The texting continued ...

Me: Liam knows I have to be back by 10.30, right?

Toby: Yes.

Me: Also, I have to inject at 7, so can't leave until after then.

My phone rang. I didn't even look at the name on the screen, it was obviously a frustrated Toby who wanted to save his texting thumb and just clarify the arrangements once and for all. But it wasn't Toby. It was a woman's voice. She might have said her name. I can't remember. After realising it was not Toby, all I recall was something like this:

'We have found suitable donor organs for you. You need to come to the ward as soon as you can, bring your bag with everything you need. You'll need to empty the dialysis fluid you have in you now. Do not panic, just get here as safely and as quickly as possible. Do you understand what I am saying?'.

I did.

Fuck fuck fuck fuck fuck fuck fuck fuck fuck fuck fuck fuck fuck.

FUUUUUUUUCK.

This was it.

I went to the bathroom and puked up whatever blandness I had just had for dinner. I called my Mum. I can't remember anything about that conversation, but I imagine, while she did not say it out loud, she probably thought the same string of expletives that I just did. She was on her way over. I threw up again.

For the rest of the evening, time meant nothing. The pamphlets the hospital had given me about this precise moment probably said what I needed to pack, and I'm sure I had read it at some point. I am sure my bag was meant to be loaded up and ready to go, like a nine month and two weeks pregnant mum-to-be with a tummy full of vindaloo. I think I put a toothbrush and some pyjama bottoms in a holdall that was probably designed for a long weekend away. I connected myself to a dialysis-draining bag and emptied my peritoneal cavity via the cursed tube, which now felt as much a part of my body as my willy did, and, in reality, was far better at draining me of fluids than 'the real thing'. It took about 20 minutes and required sitting in one place, during which time I texted and called as many people as I possibly could.

Karen was the first. It is hard to do justice to my friendship with Karen in a book which is not titled 'My friend Karen'. Our families moved into the same cul-de-sac in 1976, which for the sake of anecdotes, means I have known her since I was three years old.

FOR THE (MEDICAL) RECORD

It is not as if I've battled with mental health issues, but I've had a few minor skirmishes. Hardly my first conflict, but I was instructed to see a child psychologist by the headmaster of my first primary school. For whatever dumbfounded reason, the headmaster believed I was gifted and wanted me to be assessed as such. I'd have been about five, so have no recollection of this, but as I understand it, my mother saw this as the last straw. The school was failing anyway, so she quickly yanked me out of it. I think perhaps he mistook 'annoying' for 'gifted'.

The next confrontation came when I was in my second year of university. I don't remember sliding into a bout of depression, it was only when I slumped onto my own personal rock bottom that I realised I had made the downward-spiralling journey. It wasn't the black dog per se which alerted others to my state but rather the anorexia nervosa which accompanied it. I couldn't bring myself to eat, and if I did, I was overwhelmed by waves of nausea. My waif-like body, which was bubbling with underlying health issues, could not bear the brunt of any weight loss. By chance, I was studying emotional disorders at the time, and a liaison psychiatrist gave both counsel and cramming advice during therapy sessions. A small cabal of student housemates, who were not as hellbent on getting pissed as the others we lived with in our rancid, yet sprawling, Victorian terrace digs, sat with me evening in and evening out for months before I retreated from my funk. I only knew I was better when I was better: there were no increments of increasing happiness. I don't know where that door to the depths of my despair is located in my psyche, but I've never stumbled across it again, despite the odds stacked against my mental health well-being.

The last tussle with my mental health came in my early thirties, and I am not sure what triggered it or really what it was all about. It could've been that my father had not long been diagnosed with terminal cancer, it could have been that I had spiralling debts in the region of £10,000 after a career gear change was forced upon me, or it might have been just an identity crisis. Whatever it was, an old friend recognised in me a severe behavioural shift and recommended I went to see the counsellor that she herself had once employed the services of.

I sat in his dusty old Cambridge consulting room as he psychologically poked and probed the outer edges of my consciousness, before finding the occasional rabbit hole and jumping down it. He asked about my job (bad), my current relationship (disastrous), and he asked me about my friendships (Karen). He wasn't really that interested in her but rather the 'us' that comprised Karen and me.

I mentioned that, while we had known each other for effectively our whole lives, it was only in our teenage years that we truly bonded. Since then, while we very much have our own lives, we have been emotionally inseparable. We can, on occasion, drive each other to despair, although not in a confrontational manner, but she has always been there for me, and I like to think I've always been there for her. Halfway through talking about her, the therapist asked me to stop. He then pulled a tape recorder out, asked me if I was okay being one of his case studies, and told me to start talking about our friendship again from the start, this time with a recording device whirring away in the background. When I was done, he gave me a rather smug look, as if he had cracked the enigma code, and declared that what I had with Karen was not a 'friendship' but rather a bond akin to one experienced by twins.

He also told me that the behaviour I had recently been demonstrating put me on the sociopath spectrum, so not sure I can credit his £70 an hour opinion. I also found out later, he had given hundreds of pounds of free therapy to my friend, who was, at the time of treatment, a young and very vulnerable woman; in hindsight, that reeked of #metoo. Either way, Karen has had an immeasurable impact on my life, and I often credit her with the fact that I do not suffer from toxic masculinity, have always preferred to be in the company of women, and shudder at the very words 'a man's man'. If I was to rank friends and family by how much they fret about me, Karen is second only to my mother. During my Dialysis Days, she had made a point of calling me during every lunch break, despite the fact that she had just started a high-pressure job as a trademark attorney and probably needed any daily hour-long respite she could get. With her husband Tim, another old friend of mine, they had rallied the troops and bought me a portable DVD player for my prolonged stays in hospital. Those who contributed to the DVD player fund may not even recall donating, but I know what that now humble bit of tech meant to me. I will forever be in Karen's debt for what she has done for me.

*****

On that 2009, May 14th evening, as I furiously texted as many of my friends as I could, Karen was out in London commencing a bit of a swanky long weekend, celebrating her birthday with her husband and her family. I left a message on her voicemail, but she was at a comedy gig and had her phone turned off. Her birthday is on May 15th and buried under a wealth of emotions, I am sure she felt, upon hearing my update, that this was a typical Adrian-y way of toying with her and our bond by upstaging her birthday fun. If I had died under the knife, she might have possibly regarded it as an action of 'that'll wind her up'. As I say, our friendship has had its complications and its contradictions, but mainly it is one of compassion, caring and love.

I definitely texted Neil. He is another childhood friend, although a comparative newbie, what with me having first met him when I was ten. Neil perhaps knows me better than anyone (bar The Swedish Wife); I am never more of my natural self than when I am in his company. It was Neil who jointly picked up the mantle of responsibility when it came to ferrying me around when I was blind, on dialysis, and had two broken feet. While my mother and her partner drew the short straw with endless hospital runs, Neil – who had inherited my car – did his best to think of things to do to keep me distracted while my life ebbed away. And for a man who has an inherent disgust of all bodily functions, he was surprisingly forgiving of me as I constantly dry-heaved in the passenger seat. He'd also regularly come to my house when my vision was at its most diminished and help me with household bills, filling in forms, writing cheques and then guiding the pen to where I needed to sign.

Daniel, the most alpha of my friends, who I've known since I was five years old; Andrew, my best mate from school and later the best man at my wedding; Adrienne, a jobbing actor, and the ex I had split from just months before I received this life-changing/potentially life-ending call, and I don't know who else. I texted as many people as I could, partially because I knew they wanted to know if this news was ever to break and partially because I was scared I'd never be in contact with them ever again.

Before I knew it, my mother and Barry had arrived. If my mother's face had been any paler, it would have been translucent; meanwhile, Barry maintained a matter-of-fact, steadfast calm. He drove. Barry was well versed in the rapid pull over/emergency vomit stop, and I was au fait with much of the hedgerow which lined the laybys between my home and Addenbrookes Hospital, where I had whiled away many an hour being sick. After a quick spew stop, we parked up just outside the ward. Adrenaline had taken control of my as-near-to-death-as-it-has-so-far-gotten body, and while Barry fumbled to unfold my wheelchair, I practically sprinted gazelle-like to register my presence and claim my awaiting offal.

I was instructed to wait in a consulting room where I anxiously paced. Moments later I was joined by my mother, who was in such distress it looked like she might have witnessed some puppies being tortured in the corridor between the hospital entrance and the security door of the ward; Barry was not far behind, haplessly wielding a vacant wheelchair. My mother sat on the bed and shook with nerves. Barry, with nowhere better to plonk himself, bagsied the wheelchair. Minutes later, the surgeon, Gavin Pettigrew, arrived and introduced himself for the first time. He was casually dressed and had his trousers tucked in his socks in the manner I did as a child to prevent my trouser legs being soiled by an over-zealously oiled bicycle chain. My first thought was, *He hasn't just come from the pub, has he*? Looking at the state of us all, he would have been excused for thinking he had just wandered into a battle zone army field hospital. I was anxiously pacing, Mum looked shell-shocked and was practically vibrating with nerves on a bed, Barry appeared wheelchair-bound, like an early onset Chelsea Pensioner: 'Can I ask who I am actually operating on?' was Mr Pettigrew's justifiably bemused opening gambit.

*****

Mum, Barry, Karen, Tim, Paul, Emily, Toby, Aine, Neil, Andrew, Clare, Nick, Amy, Dan, Ally, Danny, Susana, and Helen are all headliners among the core must-visits I make when I am back in the UK.

Temporarily fast-forwarding to December 29th, 2020, and it was exactly a year since I had seen any of them. I am not cut out for not seeing these friends; I can only consider the dynamics of those relationships from my perspective, but what they did (and still do) for me plays a significant part in my feelings for them. Stoicism and stiff-upper-lipness might prevent me from writing it 'out loud', but they know what they mean to me.

A year before, on December 29th, 2019, I had woken up

in my mother's house in the home county of Essex. As per norm, the plan for me to exit the UK was to be picked up by Toby, driven to a café for a late breakfast, and then head off to the airport where, as an employee of the UK Government's Home Office, he could abuse staff parking privileges and drop me off at a relaxed pace. Hugs with Mum had been exchanged and giggles and gossip had been traded with Toby. It was a farewell like any other. No need for anyone to miss anyone to any great extent, I'd probably be back by April, at least that's normally when I need my next 'UK topping up'. But now I know that, from here on in, every farewell will be tainted and tinged with a 'what if...?'.

Spring, summer, autumn, winter – not a season goes by when I don't plonk down back on UK soil. As such a frequent visitor, my arrival prompts no fanfare. I just fit back in where I left off. I slot back in like I did the year before, the year before that, five years before then ... much in the same way I fitted in when I lived there. I haven't noticed anyone age in the eleven years I've been in Sweden. People don't have the time to wrinkle and warp within the spaces of time I don't see them. It's not just the familiarity I relish, it's a routine I cherish. But not this year. Not 2020. The first year in my life I had not seen my mother or my friends for an entire year.

We should, and rightfully so, check our privileges. Gender, race, and the bodies and minds we are born with, we have no control over, but the privilege I hold most dear are my friends, and those friendships are bolstered by the help they've given me.

*****

But rewinding back to May 2009 *and ... where the fuck were they when I needed them?!*

My guess is that it was the morning of the Saturday I had been planning to attend the quiz night, probably May 16th, 2009. The only recollection I really had of the recovery room was the *Have I shit the bed?* startling call to consciousness, but now I was in the high dependency ward and feeling abso-bloody-lutely brilliant. I was lying flat on my back, with a nurse by my side who was preoccupied with, I dunno, keeping me alive or something, and I was bored out of my mind. Did my family and friends not appreciate what I had just come through? I wanted company, conversation, chatter, and chuckles, and they were nowhere to be seen. How *dare* they!

As it later transpired, while I had spent the last two nights in an anaesthetised slumber or zonked out post-physical trauma, my two Top Fretters had not been so lucky. Karen had been booked into a fancypants hotel in Chelsea, where I imagine she was hoping to happily sleep off an evening of Michelin-starred nomming. But as it turned out, nothing puts your off your dinner and a restful sleep quite like knowing both your halibut and your best mate are soon to be filleted. Meanwhile, my mother and Barry had returned from the hospital, leaving me in the hands of Mr Pettigrew and his team, in the early hours of Friday morning (a time when those very hands would've been deep in my guts). I finally went under the knife at 3am. My mother did not sleep for the next two nights. Not a wink.

Sometime between the beginning of the Saturday and the end of the Saturday, Mum did turn up. On the Sunday, Karen and Tim visited. Word was out that I had survived, and despite having 21 tubes penetrating my body (Mum counted them while I was asleep, apparently), I was doing okay.

Me introducing Daniel as an alpha male is perhaps a little unfair. I set the bar to qualify for such derision pretty low: if you like rugby, then you are a 'probably'; if you play rugby, then you are a 'more than likely'; and if you like and play rugby and drink beer on a day that you do either, then you are 'guilty as charged'. Daniel likes sport. He is also one of the most caring and supporting friends I have. While it might be the case that when we are together, we regress to our ten-year-old selves and debate our best ever farts, Daniel is nevertheless one of the most stable and together people I know. And that stability affords him the luxury of helping others, in this case (but not exclusively), me. While he has a demanding job, which involves late nights and travel, he was always there, at the other end of the phone, ready to pick up prescriptions and groceries and answer any whim my diseased body required.

By the Monday, I had been moved to a room that I shared with a man who had just had a kidney transplant, and his brother-in-law, who had just donated him his kidney. We had all just left the high dependency so were placed near the nurses' station due to our precarious, but now stable, states. I was woken from a doze by a familiar voice coming from outside the room; it was a man asking where Adrian was. 'Is he the patient who has recently donated one of his kidneys?' the nurse asked.

'I fucking well hope not. His don't work', said the man. The familiar voice was Daniel's. He took one look at me and told me I looked like crap, and I could not have been happier to see anyone. Not one for kid gloves, at least not around me, it did not take us long to get back to a scatological-themed, poo-peppered conversation, and I had so much to tell him. Normality was starting to resume.

Over the next week or so, while I underwent physio, rehab and carried out an apparently unnoticed charm offensive on Pharmacy Girl, all my favourite people visited. All brought different qualities to the table/bedside. Barry, my mother's partner, for example, is more of a logistics man. When it comes to someone else's decrepit adult son, he prefers a supporting yet vital role. When we left my house with my poorly packed bag and a blended sense of dread and relief, I was painfully aware I was leaving my full-time companion behind me. Milo the Bastard was a tabby cat who had been with/tolerated me through every phase of my ill health. I might have hated those dialysis boxes, but he, however, quite enjoyed sleeping in them. Had he been able to speak, and I told him I was about to leave for three weeks for life saving surgery, he probably would have helped me pack, suggested I left for four weeks ('to be on the safe side') and then suggested I leave my keys ('just in case the worst happens'). If I had returned 20 minutes later, realising I had forgotten my phone charger, I'd have been greeted with a 'where-the-hell-have-you-been?' death stare. As much fickle as he was feral – that cat. And Barry was there for his every beck and call – and bite and scratch – in my absence.

As it turned out, I couldn't have done a worse job of packing for a hospital stay. I didn't need a toothbrush because all my dietary requirements were provided via a tube and judging by how far down my transplant scars go and the botched manscaping job of my pubes I woke up with, none of the surgeon's team slipped me into my jim-jams as part of the pre-op/post-anaesthetic procedures. Within a week, Barry was instructed to find a few t-shirts from a chest of drawers while he was checking in with Milo the Bastard.

I am not quite sure how he managed it, but I can only presume he chose to pluck t-shirts from the back of the drawer with the logic that these were the ones I used the least and were therefore probably the most suitable attire while my whole body was a bit 'leaky'. However, what he had unwittingly chosen was one band t-shirt with a very large tombstone on it, and another which featured the word 'fuck' on it. Both t-shirts were from my youth and certainly not suitable for a ward full of people who were fresh out of major surgery. Barry went back to my house to get more; I think he was probably using it as an excuse to spend more time with Milo.

*****

And so my care continued (and continues). Despite my outward-facing appearance of being a grownup with a job, The Swedish Wife, my family, and my friends provide much of the scaffolding to construct this illusion. After I was discharged, Barry continued with logistical support, offering countless lifts to the hospital for follow-up appointments and blood tests. And, seeing as I was forbidden to bathe with my still-stapled-up scar and the fact that my home did not have a shower, Daniel would fetch me every Saturday morning, let me use his en suite bathroom and then redress my fast-healing wounds in scenes akin to a homoerotic remake of *The English Patient.*

But, from 2020 and onwards, help has never been in such high demand, and while I can only speak for myself, it is important for people to know how appreciated help, in all its guises, can be. Many of my friends and family covered more than just one help base, but Karen certainly ticked The Caller box in relation to help needed. We've been neighbours, lived just one village away, and even been housemates, but when I was at my sickest we lived over a hundred miles apart. At this time, she was my most frequent caller, hence her status as a Caller and not a Pop-Inner. At that time, pre-transplant, when she was calling the most, my iron levels were rapidly depleting, and despite having more than one blood transfusion and a regular self-administered shot of erythropoietin (or 'EPO' as it is known by winning, albeit cheating, Tour de France cyclists), I was putting Milo the Bastard cat to shame when it came to sleeping all day. Karen would call and I would want to answer, but sometimes I was just too tired or too weak. My phone would ring, and I would panic. I was just so used to calls during office hours from doctors delivering the next set of devastating blood test results. So increasingly I'd see her name appear on my screen and ignore it, just relieved it was not a 'we need to admit you' call. But I was always happy to know she was thinking of me. So never underestimate your role as a Caller, even if your calls go unanswered.

Pop-Ins were few and far between in the UK. Most of my friends worked full time and selfishly prioritised looking after their kids over me, but when they happened, they stood out from the Pick-Uppers. Pop-Ins were always of a social nature and would normally centre around watching a film rented en route to my abode. Of late, Pandemic Pop-Ins were held in my apartment block's shared garden. Pick-Uppers were, of course, essential, but this normally meant another trip to the hospital; Mum was the most frequent Pick-Upper, but Barry was used for emergencies when Mum's nerves were too rattled and speed was of the essence.

Ill health is not a luxury lifestyle choice, but it sure has its expenses. There were times when I was reliant on public transport, there were times when I travelled courtesy of hospital transport, but there were many, many times when my life depended on taxis, the fare for which was footed by my mother, who so often had to escort me. She, among so many other help roles, became The Benefactor. It did not matter how disabled-friendly train stations were, how many ramps and lifts could elevate me to my destination, there were many occasions when the only way from home to hospital was by taxi. My mother's pension pot was depleted by this 'luxury'. Sometimes we could claim the fare back from the authorities, sometimes we couldn't. Whatever the case, this took its toll on my mother's life savings.

But this is not solely a homage to my friends and family in the UK. In Sweden, The Helpers among my friends quickly drew themselves to my attention. will&brandy, our neighbours, as they appear on my list of nearby Wi-Fi networks, were well aware that it was not about helping just me but rather our household. Tess, who had shrugged off Covid like a loose-fitting cashmere cardigan, obviously did not need protecting, but the logic was (before we actually got it, at least), that Tess putting herself at risk would ipso facto put me at risk. will&brandy were never more than a WhatsApp message away and performed any delivery we required with military precision. On a number of occasions, they assumed the role of The Benefactors with a just-buy-us-a-drink-when-this-is-all-over   philanthropic mentality. Former colleague-cum-pal, Janni, armed with the experience of living with someone who overlaps my condition (although I'd win at Transplant Top Trumps, as he's only a kidney transplant recipient), has always fought – or at least padded – my corner in a world of unwitting and unknowing ableists.

Much help is received under the guise of friendship, but that is certainly not exclusively the case. There have been times when my blood pressure has yo-yoed to extremes, and I've 'come over all a bit wobbly'. In both the UK and Sweden, total randos have raced to the conclusion that I should sit down, not assuming I am drunk or high on crack, but rather that this is a medical emergency, mild or otherwise. Random Help is not, in my humble opinion, as prevalent as it could be, but I like to think it is on the up – if you ain't a Random Helper already, join their ranks now. But I am not just a helpée, while my instinct might come from nature, nurture has played its role; being the recipient of so much help has certainly made me understand its value and pay it forward.

I know I demand more than I supply, but I can't see a time when, globally, help is not a sought-after commodity – it can be found in bottomless pits – never stop thinking it is not needed or appreciated. Never stop helping.

FOR THE (MEDICAL) E-RECORD

Those who feel the need to vocally defend their excessive use of social media tend to cite such reasons as shyness, remoteness, disability, something about cats, dick pics, a need for a vital communication tool for the logistical demands of distributing aid to disaster-struck regions, or the overthrowing of a ruthless despot.

On the occasion that a tech blip shuts down an entire platform – or indeed platforms – some will scoff at users, believing that communication tools such as Facebook Messenger and Twitter are used for nothing but trifling tosh.

I beg to differ. Both in sickness and in health, social media has done nothing but enhance my life; without it, I would have neither a wife nor a job.

I am fortunate enough to have 'real life' friends from when I was growing up ('Village Friends'), school friends, university friends, college friends, work friends, friends of friends, and now, Swedish friends. But thrown into that heady mix are online friends – online friends who have become 'real life' friends and 'real life' friends who are now just online friends.

And Michelle.

I met Michelle on Myspace, the social network platform which dominated while Mark Zuckerberg was still wanking in his dorm room over photos submitted to Facemash, the 'hot or not' photo comparison website which would later evolve into Facebook.

Michelle and I had/have a lot in common. Our messages were good humoured and filled with day-to-day trivialities and candid details of our respective dating endeavours. She lived 'up North', and I was a 'southern softie', but beyond the distance divide, we seemed to have an unwritten agreement to never meet IRL (in real life). We are still in sporadic contact to this day but have only spoken a handful of times.

When I was first admitted to hospital for potential kaput kidneys – when Professor Edmonds had called me out of the blue on that Sunday afternoon – I was thrown under, on, in and through every scanning device the hospital had a working plug for.

'Hey, Michelle, it's Adrian from Myspace. I don't have brain cancer' were my first spoken words to Michelle. I am not sure why she was first to hear this news. She just was. I didn't think I had brain cancer in the first place, but the doctors wanted to rule it out, and I thought this particular result from this particular machine would make for a fun opening conversation starter.

In 2009, six years after we became Myspace friends and were still in regular contact, I was sitting up in bed. It was a week after the transplant, and my mother had come to visit, bringing with her some get well cards. The most memorable one being from Beth, another internet friend. She had sent me a card designed for someone who had just passed their driving test. 'Congratulations! You've passed' read the caption, after which Beth had written in biro, 'urine'.

Along with the cards was a parcel, in which was a beautifully wrapped box containing a silver hallmarked hip flask. Squished in next to it was a small bottle of vodka. 'I always wanted to smuggle some booze into a hospital', was Michelle's texted justification for this gift. The flask, today, sits in my most-treasured items drawer.

At the time, Michelle had a friend who worked in pharmaceutical research. She put me in touch with her, and this complete stranger, who knew nothing of me other than my health predicament, guided me through the ins, outs and every possible side effect of the drugs I was being loaded with.

So when it comes to defending social media use, I talk

about my wife, Tess, and how I got my job, Patrick. If that's not enough, there's no better further justification than Michelle.

The pandemically enforced travel restrictions, which at first were self-imposed, but then just a part of a global reality, hit me hard. I had gone from restraining myself from seeing my UK friends in the early stages of the pandemic to being restricted from seeing them. Now what else could the world have thrown at me to further divide me from the people who have helped me the most?

Chapter 12
Bloody, shitty immigrants (my blood, my shit)

Of course – Brexit. I had forgotten all about Brexit.

It was difficult, wasn't it? Knowing which body part you were supposed to employ to help decide which box you ticked in the 2016 EU referendum. And it was hard to fathom which body part meant what. If you were thinking with your heart, for example, were you being a 'loyal subject of the crown, a patriot, and a supporter of sovereignty'? Or were you using that same organ to consider the plight of future generations or those who sought to better their lives with no more than a one-way trip on a budget airline? Perhaps you were thinking with your head, and after a night of sherry-fuelled number crunching, with calculations written with a fountain pen on a parchment-themed notepad your son-in-law Barnaby got you for a 'jolly' Christmas gift and using a copy of Adam Smith's *The Wealth of Nations* as 'something to lean on', quite genuinely believed that leaving the EU would be a fiscal advantage to the UK. Alternatively, you might've used your head and carried out the calculations we all learned in primary school with an abacus to do some tariff totting-up and times tables, and within 45 seconds, easily concluded that leaving the EU would leave the UK financially fucked.

I decided to base my decision on a completely different part of my body, namely my bottom. Well, not my bottom per se, but rather a night in May 2009 when I shit my bed. A bed shitting which did not shift my heartfelt and deeply entrenched political beliefs, but certainly one which reinforced them.

The bed in question was a hospital bed. While I had had the phantom fear that I'd soiled my sheets just a week earlier after waking from transplant surgery, this, like an infinitely better-marketed brown liquid, was 'the real thing'. It was during my second week of being a convalescing inpatient, and the pain control that had been keeping me in that perpetual state of feeling abso-bloody-lutely fantastic had found a new agony to contend with.

I had now been writhing in pain for days, and if there is one thing I know all about, it is pain. On the one-to-ten agony scale, I've experienced every digit on the gauge in excruciating, brutal, analogue detail. Loitering on the steps to Death's Door does bring all manner of hurts, but none, none so great, as I now know, as trapped wind. Yip, gas. What is fart to you, was purgatory for me. Blinding migraines, nerve-wracked neuropathic pain, and even that time the sedatives wore off and I woke up mid operation: I've felt more than I should have on the spectrum of pain. But nothing, nothing comes close to trapped wind.

So there I was, lying in a ward having just days earlier had a team of doctors playing with my innards with – what now felt like – all the grace of an exploratory delve into a fairground lucky dip. Food was being pumped into me, but my twisted and tangled intestines were insisting that none of it was to pass. A number of days and nights went by when a wheeled commode was rushed to my bedside at my urgent request, but alas, nothing. It was the same for the other two patients I shared the room with. One evening, a loud fart was met with rapturous applause and cheers of congratulations for the patient whose guts had eased just enough to allow a puff of wind through. If he could do it, then perhaps there was hope for the rest of us.

Then, one night, a sudden-start to a slow realisation. The pumped food had found an out and made a bolt for it. I was lying in a pool of my own despicable making. Emergency buzzer pressed, and two nurses, fully attired in disposable aprons and latex gloves, came to my rescue and went to task. 'I'm sorry', I pleaded to one of them, as she wet and dry wiped the epicentre of the disaster zone before moving down the back of my legs. She continued her meticulous scrubbing, onto my ankles and then my feet – my deformed, shit-splattered feet.

'It's okay, it's my job', she politely insisted in a noticeable foreign accent. 'But it can't be your favourite part of the job', I randomly reasoned. 'Where are you from?' I added, in a bid to move the conversation into slightly more civil territory. 'Greece', came the response, as she went to help the other nurse change the soiled bed sheets. The acrid smell of festering poo mixed in with internally bled blood left a metallic funk in the air, the tang of iron hit my taste buds prompting a kneejerk vomit.

The other nurse came to my aid, and my previous conversation apparently duplicated itself. 'Romania', she answered. And with my bottom in mind, there I pondered what a Brexited immigration point system could bring. Sure, we might be able to cherry-pick the researchers, the doctors, and the professors, but could our vital services survive without the carers and the cleaners? Could we afford to shut out our continental neighbours who come to the UK to better their lives by bettering our lives?

*****

I can't say it was at the top of my mind as I sat with Tess at 11pm on 31st December 2020, when the transition period ended, and the UK, under the cover of darkness, severed itself, once and for all, from the EU. At that precise time, while we felt like we had cleared the Covid hurdle which had blighted our Christmas just a week earlier, I can't say that we were in a particularly celebratory frame of mind. We were both hyper-sensitive when it came to any sniff, throat tickle or cough – both of us still uncertain whether we had successfully evicted the spiky little virus from our home. Hardly the best set of circumstances to celebrate New Year's Eve, and the icing on the cake – or the coulis on the venison, in this case – was that Tess could still only taste and smell the occasional whisp of garlic from her gourmet cooking labours.

I had actually been a Swedish citizen for over a year at this point. I am not sure if it was by pure coincidence or the impish sense of humour of a Swedish government administrator, but the confirmation of my dual nationality arrived in the post on 29th March 2019 – the original end of the Article 50 period and the first, but bungled, planned date for Brexit. Waking up in Sweden on New Year's Day 2021, nothing had noticeably changed, I felt the same as I did when the Millennium Bug was set to destroy civilisation in planes-falling-from-the-skies scenes only previously witnessed in Hollywood disaster B movies. And I would have imagined that in the UK the bananas were still the same shape and English and French fishermen were still slapping each other around the face with wet cod, disputing which bits of the La Manche/the English Channel (delete as applicable) they could each deplete and destroy.

But what of those two nurses? Where are they now? Highly skilled nurses working in a transplant ward. Nurses who could wrap their brains around the state-of-the-art gizmos keeping me alive one minute and then be on their knees scrubbing my puke and poo off the floor before guiding me to a wheelchair commode the next. They had, after all, worked the machines which fed me, so they probably had a fairly good idea of how much there was yet to come out of me. They can't be the easiest people to replace if they decided to up sticks and leave, right?

Hospital porters though? Possibly perceived – by those who have no idea how every cog is vital – as being at the bottom of the hospital food chain. I doubt they'd make the grade for any points-based immigration policy ...

FOR THE (MEDICAL) RECORD

I knew I was feeling poorly. My head felt like a glass orb, and even an eyeball swivel would cause a lightning-strike fork of pain into the centre of my brain. Apart from that, it felt like a non-descript Sunday afternoon. It was July 2008, just under a year before I was to have transplant surgery (not that I knew this at the time). I was waiting to be picked up from my home so I could spend the afternoon and early evening with my mother, a slight respite from my own four walls. When making that arrangement, I had re-layed a selection of symptoms which were currently blight-ing me, and unbeknown to me, or at least my recollections, Mum had called for medical advice. Before I knew it, my mum and Barry had arrived, and I was being bundled into a car like a hostage and driven with a determined speed towards casualty. I knew I was feeling poorly, but I had no idea how poorly until I witnessed the response from the accident and emergency crew upon my arrival.

Within minutes I was lying on a gurney and surrounded by a team of doctors and nurses who were running every test on every machine they had in their vicinity. And that vicinity had more machines than the flight deck of the *Starship Enterprise*. Cannulas were pinned into my veins, giving ready access to blood, and tubes were shoved down my nose giving ready access to ... I don't know, whatever is down there. Despite being in what felt like a scene from a hospital drama, the staff all laboured away with a calm steadfast and measured determination. In fact, I only heard one raised and tinkering-on-the-brink-of-anger voice. The anger, however, was not directed at me. It came from a doctor who was talking on the phone to what I can only assume was the hospital's bed manager. He had heard that there were no beds available on the kidney ward, to which his response was, along the sentiment of, whoever is the least urgent patient in that ward, get them out – 'We have a man in casualty who needs that bed'. That man was me. As I said, I knew I was feeling poorly.

The reason the doctor was being so uppity was because he had concluded I was suffering from ketoacidosis, and unlike me, he didn't need Google to understand its life-threatening nature or identify the symptoms of vomiting, abdominal pain, deep-gasping breathing, increased urination, weakness, confusion and occasionally loss of consciousness. Or 'feeling poorly', as I wrote in the first place.

I was wheeled to the ward where I ended up staying for the next ten days. The condition was basically caused by a non-compliant pancreas, and all I really remember from a medical recovery perspective was a lot of sleep and a blood transfusion. But what I will definitely never forget is the patient in the bed next to me.

I never once spoke to him. Firstly, because I was too ill to maintain any form of coherent conversation beyond answering the questions of medical staff; and secondly, because he did not speak a word of English. I couldn't help but eavesdrop into the healthcare professionals' conversations though, and from what I could gather, his current lifestyle was best described as 'chaotic'. He was, from what I understood, overly partial to a bit of a tipple, and on top of the booze, he might regularly participate in certain opiate-based narcotic recreational pursuits.

I felt incredible sympathy for this individual. He looked worse for wear and possibly beyond being patched up, but for all I know, he was looking across from his bed, vacantly gazing at me and thinking to himself, *Jezu, co się z nim stało?*. It was of deep frustration to the medical staff doing the morning rounds, that a translator was always required to communicate anything but the basics of his possible road to recovery. There were definitely mutterings of how many qualified and procured interpreters they had access to, and from what I could garner, there was only one woman covering the region who always seemed to be available, albeit a two hours' drive away at the point of asking for her services.

So this patient, from Poland as it came to light, would communicate through a series of points, head nods, and headshakes until the interpreter arrived and the more complicated details of his medical condition could be explained. That was the way it was, until two particular porters arrived. Polish porters. It didn't take them long to clock one of their countryfolk, and friendly glances were soon being exchanged. At one point, the patient motioned one of the passing porters over and engaged in a more protracted Polish conversation. Later, when both the porters were in earshot and communicating in English, the subject of what was raised in the earlier conversation was discussed. One agreed to pass on some details to a member of the medical staff. Not long after, a doctor swished closed the curtain which divided us. He was with the patient for quite some time.

I don't know for sure what was relayed from the patient, via the porter, to the doctor, or whether the porters were pivotal to the patient's treatment. What I do know is this, not many porters who have been through the UK education system are multilingual, capable code-switchers. Like the nurses, those porters can't be the easiest people to replace if they decided to up sticks and leave, right?

*****

Rarely do I note the colour, creed, or country of birth of any medical practitioner that has treated me over the years. The Hippocratic Oath is recognised pretty much globally, and that's all that really matters to me. There was a time when I was being given a kidney ultrasound by a woman with the thickest, southern states of America drawl I'd heard since watching the Dukes of Hazzard and drooling over Daisy Duke. I definitely remember commenting on that – it practically sounded otherworldly. She was from Alabama and had decided to spend a year in London. There was also a time when I noticed that all five doctors standing around my bed who were taking it in turns to read my case file were either Indian or of Indian descent. One of them had been one of my regular checker-uppers and was keen to introduce the others – all junior to him but on the same medical career trajectory to reach his dizzying heights of academic achievement. And the only thought which sprang to mind was, where on earth would the National Health Service be without the waves of immigration the UK has done nothing but benefit from? Beyond those, I can only think of one other occasion the heritage of a doctor was ever raised ...

It was April 2010, still less than a year since my transplant, and the man on the other side of the desk was describing to me, in brutal detail, how he was planning to carve up my cock, and he was doing it with a funny accent. Well, not funny, just an accent I could not for the life of me place. Perhaps I should have been concentrating a little more on the subject at hand, bearing in mind he was fully engrossed in the graphic depiction of the disposal of a bit of my body he felt was surplus to requirements but that I had always been rather fond of. Still, my foreskin was for the chop, and I think, truth be told, we both knew it was for the best. Still, funny accent.

'That's an interesting accent', I said, diplomatically. 'Can I ask where you are from?' I didn't care that much, obviously, but could we just change the penis-themed conversation, even just for a while? He bit.

'I bet you can't even guess. You'll never get it', he jovially challenged. He was up for this. Did he have a Mediterranean complexion? Possibly, but he didn't sound Italian, Greek, or Spanish. Maybe Middle Eastern, my crappy vision was doing me no favours with this guessing game.

'Syrian?', I cautiously proposed. He rolled his eyes and, almost triumphantly responded, 'Way off. Try again'. I really didn't have a clue, and his eagerness to play this game was kind of freaking me out a little. I guess he might've been Asian. I threw a wild card out there, partly because, despite previously wanting respite from the topic, I now wanted to bring this conversation back to my genitals and partly because I might just have been right.

'Thailand?'

He laughed. 'I am from Cyprus'. And he was clearly very proud of the fact, judging by how he steered the conversation to his family history. He now evidently wanted to talk more about where his great grandparents were from rather than chatting about slicing my willy in two, which, under any other circumstances, would have been completely fine, but I was getting anxious and just wanted to get this appointment done and dusted – I was regretting my decision to probe. For the record, the doctor, from my then local surgery who referred me to this consultant, was South African.

Obviously, some of these 'case studies' were, in theory, not going to be affected by Brexit, but what about the nationalist sentiments the referendum debate stirred-up? Time will tell. Personally, I thought I had dodged the Brexit Bullet by being the owner of both an in-the-EU and an out-of-the-EU passports. Turns out that was not to be the case.

*****

I've never described myself as an 'expat', purely on the grounds that I was never a 'pat' in the first place. And instinctively, I never use the word 'Blighty', as in 'I am heading back to Blighty for the weekend'. I just can't disassociate it from leathery-skinned Boomers complaining about the full English breakfasts they're wolfing down in the Costa del Sol: 'We need to get back to Blighty, Shirley. You can't get a decent banger or a cuppa 'ere', et cetera. And it turns out my instinct has served me well, cursory Wiki-knowledge informs me the word 'Blighty' derives from Bengali. It originally meant 'English visitor' and came about during Britain's blood-drenched rule of India – that hardly adds favour to the word. It was first used as a nostalgic reference to Britain as a homeland while British troops were once again shooting up the place in South Africa in the late 19th Century. Britain will never be 'Blighty' to me. When I return there, it is not uncommon for me to simply say, 'I am going back to Mum's'.

There seemed to be much talk of identity during the run-up to the referendum debate. Some, very much in the Leave camp, were keen to nationalistically pin their colours to the English flag bearing the Saint George Cross. An ilk with a penchant for joining the far-right-wing English Defence League and proudly boasting, 'I am English 'til I die'. Meanwhile, the liberal elite, *Guardian* reader types, with far more of a Remain rhetoric, might claim, 'I am European' or 'I am a citizen of the World'. While politically I sympathise with the latter, I have to confess that just like the former, I identify as being English.

But to qualify the comment and quash the criticism, I am far from being the type to march down a street with a bunch of neo-Nazis chanting 'There ain't no black, there ain't no black, there ain't no black in the Union Jack' (my eyesight is too cloudy to identify what colours are in any flag, truth be told). If I happen to be marching down the same street at the same time, you'll very much find me marching in the opposite direction. To my self-deprecating mind, however, I just can't imagine that any other nation would want me identifying with them. I've hardly ever been to Wales and Scotland, and I've never visited Northern Ireland – who am I to identify with any country other than the one I was born in? Especially countries we've historically ruled thanks to bludgeoning and bullying. Anything else just seems presumptuous and arrogant to me. I am nowhere near suave, stylish, chic, or sophisticated enough to get away with saying 'I am European'. Anyone living on the continent's mainland would look upon my overly-apologetic, bumbling and awkward self and say 'Non non, you iz nat wan av os', quite probably in an accent which would sound like they were trying to seduce me.

Fortunately, I rarely have to say where I am from, and the only time I really ever have to admit my nationality is on a form where they have failed to offer the option of 'I'd rather not say'. Even bearing all that in mind, when I was growing up, I'd be playfully teased by my family elders with the taunt, 'You can't be British!'. The reason? I didn't drink tea.

FOR THE (MEDICAL) RECORD

Sometime after my transplant surgery in 2009, I was offered scant details regarding the previous (apparently very careful and then, all of a sudden, very careless) owner of my new organs. He was a he, and he was 19 years old. That's all I know, and probably all I will ever know. I was invited to write a letter to his family, which I duly did, albeit over a year after the surgery and just months before I was set to move to Sweden. I didn't want to write to the family if I had rejected their loved one's organs in the first year, lest they think I was trying to claim new ones from one of his siblings under a warranty agreement they had signed in the grief-stricken aftermath of his death.

The letter protocol is as follows: the organ recipient is asked by a transplant coordinator at the hospital where the surgery took place if they'd like to write a letter. You can then choose whether you'd like to write a letter or not (you are not given the option to email, text, or send a WhatsApp message using only emojis). There is no pressure. The letter is handed over to the coordinator, who then contacts a member of staff at the hospital where the organs were plucked from the donor. That person then contacts the family and informs them that a letter has been marked for their attention. It is then up to the deceased's nearest and dearest to decide whether they want to read it, and, if they choose to do so, whether they wish to respond. As I have never received a reply, I cannot say if they have even read it. That'd be a shame, as it really was a very nice letter in my bestest and neatest handwriting, and it took me bloody days to write.

*****

Among the world of the transplanted, where some of the survivors of such ill health thank Jesus and not the surgeon and use the word 'miracle' rather than 'education', can lie the notion that the soul or spirit of the deceased may somehow live and linger on in its new host. Even my own friends have asked me if I think the deceased has partly morphed into my flesh. And that notion was always raised when it was noticed that I now drink tea. I had, up to the point I was spliced, never in my life drunk a cup of tea. And yet here I now am, a regular tea chugger.

Sadly, for the fantasists, the truth is rather mundane. When I reappeared from consulting rooms after countless appointments in the years preceding the transplant, I'd find my mum thousand-yard-staring into what I suspect was a dystopic plight for her son. I'd have left the room zapped of energy and will, and she'd often be cradling a lukewarm cup of milky, sweet tea in one of those overly squishy vended plastic cups. I'd take a sip just to wet my dehydrated lips. Everything about that one sip was strictly off-limits due to my dietary restrictions, thus, at the time, a drink that had only ever disgusted me now tasted like the elixir of the gods.

Forward-wind two days after my transplant surgery, and I braved my first hot drink, a cup of coffee. The inside of my throat was red raw from the tubes it had had rammed down it during the surgery, and the coffee felt like gravel. I took one gulp and gave up. 'How about a milky tea?' the nurse doing the drinks round suggested. She even encouraged me to have sugar, as I needed all the calories I could get. So maybe in that moment I became just a little bit more British, although, for all I know, the 19-year-old man I had now partly engulfed was an international student from China, and what do the Chinese drink in abundance? Who knows, maybe he does live on in me after all. And that possible language barrier would certainly help explain why his family never responded to my letter.

*****

There were certainly somethings which never came up on any referendum pamphlet or manifesto. Whether you were a Take-Back-Control Leaver, or a Better-Together Remainer, one thing you were never asked to consider was flight restrictions during a global pandemic, or, for that matter, what happens to the country you might just buy most of your flat-pack furniture from if your country buys up all the personal protection equipment and pre-orders three times the amount of vaccine that it actually needs. It's always the little things you forget, eh? Boris Johnson and all his cronies seemed very proud of the fact that, now out of the EU, they could use their fifth biggest economy in the world status to buy infinitely too much of what was most in demand during the pandemic before its European neighbours could. From where I was sitting in Sweden (not on an IKEA chair, FYI), it just seemed like political point scoring. The fact that one of the NHS nurses who kept vigil by the PM's side while he himself was in intensive care with Covid later resigned due to his handling of the pandemic says it all, really. She was born in New Zealand, and by all accounts went back there.

And while those in the UK were favouring what they referred to as the 'Oxford vaccine', thinking it was the Best of British and developed by an eccentric-looking geek who plays croquet with his chums at the weekend, please remember its full name is 'Oxford–AstraZeneca COVID-19 vaccine'. AstraZeneca is a British–Swedish company, founded in 1999 during the heady days of the EU. It's top bod at the time of writing, for the record, is a Swede.

So while the 'Leave the EU' campaign shot itself in the foot and sustained an injury that would require a now-drained-of-staff NHS to treat, it also, for a big chunk of the pandemic, with its shape-shifting travel restrictions, made it a damn sight harder for me to see my family and friends. And I'll never forgive the Leavers for that.

Chapter 13
'VD' stands for 'Vaccination Day'

Never before had I felt so compelled to question my marriage, although I am not really sure why I hadn't already done so. Seeds of doubt sprout and bloom very easily in my mind, and on a handful of occasions, loosely acquainted friends had told me there was something 'not quite right' about mine and Tess's relationship. The remarks were made when I had fleetingly referred to some machinations of our marriage, normally in Tess's absence.

It was a year into the pandemic when it occurred to me that, while we were far from unique, there was something which made a few ponder our suitability. Tess, AKA The Swedish Wife, and I have lived together since 2010 and took our vows in 2013. The wedding ceremony took less than one minute, and the registrar who oversaw the formalities had cycled to the outdoor location, slung her bike up against a tree, and performed the service without even removing her small daypack from her shoulders. Neither of us is big on ceremonies, nor vows, so this suited us just fine. If I'd thought getting married would have had one iota of an impact on my life, I wouldn't have agreed to the commitment.

There is, quite certainly, a fair amount we don't have in common. She reacts to my taste in music very much in the manner my father did when hearing the 'infernal din' coming from my teenage bedroom. In echoes of my formative years, Tess pleads with me, 'Can you turn that racket down? I can't even hear myself think. How on earth can *that* be described as music?' You get the picture. And while we both enjoy flomping on the sofa in the evening, it can take some lengthy debate before we finally agree on the next telly boxset to invest our 'binge time' into – I'll suggest a trending series, and Tess will veto anything which doesn't feature animals and/or dragons.

(Tess's moniker of 'The Swedish Wife', for the record, came about after a good-natured conversation we had regarding my serial monogamous dating history. Prior to Tess, I had gone out with a Frenchwoman, a Croat, an American and a Belgian. 'How do I know I am not just another one of your international girlfriends?' she questioned. 'Because they were girlfriends ... you are my wife. You're The Swedish Wife', was my cack-mouthed and borderline chauvinistic retort, and the first-recorded use of this now-familiar pet name. I further thwarted her fears by suggesting that a partially sighted metrosexual with the physique of a stick of celery and the apparent compulsion to apologise for his very existence would make for a rather farcical 'international man of mystery'.

Tess and I would flippantly laugh off any suggestion there was something odd about our pairing. Not that anyone ever said it directly to us, but rather it was always inferred, and it was normally prompted by the counter-intuitive theory that 'there is something wrong with couples who don't argue'. Such a peculiar logic. I've even heard people remark that there is something distinctly unhealthy about couples who don't have a regular clear-the-air fight. It probably doesn't help our cause that – and once again, I'll never quite fathom this – we have implicit trust in each other. So, if I happen to have dinner with a female friend – who by chance is single and, in the eyes of the shallow-minded, conforms to a conventional aesthetic of beauty – it is only a matter of time before a friend or colleague will suggest that Tess must be mad. Likewise, if I were to mention to the same crowd that Tess was to go out with a group of male colleagues, I'd be met with a warning of, 'C'mon, you know what men are like?!' Well, yes I do, and most, but certainly not all, are complete twats, but I know and trust Tess better. And that's what really matters.

Weird we live in a world where a cohabiting couple who don't argue and who implicitly trust each other are considered the anomaly. Weirder still, if one is to apply that logic, that as the pandemic ploughed on into 2021, statistics revealed divorce, trial separation, domestic violence and femicide were the aftereffects of spending increased time with the person you purportedly love the most. Turns out that the vow of 'until death us do part' should probably be amended to 'until we have to live with each other 24/7'. Meanwhile, our occasionally questioned relationship remained undinted.

With it just being the two of us – unimpeded by any offspring – working from home quickly proved to be a more productive approach to getting stuff out of your inbox than working from work. Go figure. And while I often deliver a what-the-fuck raised eyebrow in Tess's direction as she permits our cat Ogden to tongue-polish his nether regions on the dining table, I can't imagine that the stress is equivalent to finding out your 13-year-old son is using the newly-set-up-in-pandemic-haste digital teaching platform to sext his German teacher. Tess worked in one room, and I worked in another. On occasion, we'd find ourselves both making a cup of coffee at the same time, and unlike sanctioned office environments, it was okay to playfully slap one another's arses as we passed.

Around February 2021, the UK vaccine rollout was going just as fast as the grannies and granddads could be rolled into vaccination centres. Sweden, and the rest of the EU, was not far behind, but despite my vulnerable predicament, I can quite honestly say that I felt no inherent rush to fold up my sleeve and get spiked. Not a sentiment loaded with anti-vax bullshit but rather one from … I am not really too sure, but I guess the 'new normal' overlapped with my 'as near-to-utopia' as my reality was ever going to get. I had become a working-from-home evangelist, finding myself both more productive with my workload and far more protected from my potentially infected workmates.

Pre-new normal, I never really suffered from FOMO, but I am a sucker for accepting invites out of politeness rather than any real desire to attend. The new normal was lending itself to intimate, yet safely spaced 1-2-1 meetups rather than group get-togethers; I thrive in the former and, due to nothing but my disabilities, am socially thwarted by the latter.

*****

Quite when my aversion to large social gatherings started I don't really know, but it wasn't just a question of becoming a boring old bastard – far from it. The events, there were two, that sealed the deal, and why I'll happily and readily never attend another party again, are ineradicably etched onto my psyche. Both the events happened post-transplant, both happened in Sweden, and both are related to hidden disabilities, ableism, and Swedish etiquette quirks. And there is not a single (social) crutch which can help me.

Before moving to Sweden, the last time I was requested to take off my shoes before entering someone's home was probably when I was around ten years old and my friend's parents had just bought a spanking new shagpile carpet for their hallway and living room. When I was ten, it was taken as red that I'd leave a trail of traipsed mud wherever I went. But, as an adult, one can reasonably assume that any guest entering your home for dinner or a social occasion has not come straight from a playing field where they've been mucking around with their mates and making bows and arrows from sticks and string. In Sweden, apparently, that assumption is not made. The first thing any guest does upon entering any home is de-shoe. Every hallway has a shoe rack with ample space for the footwear of friends, and a shoehorn close at hand to hasten the re-shoeing process. Muscle memory kicks in once over the threshold and the Average Swede's brain, on apparent autopilot, reaches down to one-by-one shed their footwear.

My feet progressively and noticeably deformed themselves from around 2002 onwards. With every new bump and lump came newly shaped, supportive orthotics. My skeletal structure has been roundabouts stable from circa 2008, and in regard to running off to join the circus as a travelling freak, the remains of the Elephant Man would still beat me to the headline spot (deformed) hands down. But keeping those lumps and bumps in check, however, does come with a host of medical directives. Top of that list? Never walk barefoot or in socks on any surface, ever.

One becomes aware of this Swedish shoe etiquette societal norm quickly. When I was first visiting Tess and, subsequently, her family, I was excused on medical grounds, but that's because they were on a steep learning curve as to the nature of my disabilities.

I am rather tickled by the image that every Saturday night in Sweden, there will be thousands of people spending hours preening and pruning and getting ready to head out to a friend or relative's home for a drinks and dinner party. They'll be pulling out various combinations from wardrobes: Does that blouse go with this skirt? Does this jacket go with these shoes? No matter the effort and the coordinated combinations, the minute they arrive at their destination, they'll be plodding around in their socks or stockings for the rest of the evening, all because the hosts will naturally assume their guests made a game of seeing how much dog shit they could tread in en route to the soirée.

So, these are my choices when faced with the de-shoeing quandary: number one, I risk taking my shoes off and hope I'll be able to sit down a few hobbled steps away from where I've left them. This option is rife with social awkwardness unless the majority of the people in the room are aware of my feet faults. When making a beeline for the first chair available, I just look rude, particularly if most others are still standing and mingling. The second option is to bring my orthotic sandals with me; this is by far the best for my feet but will invariably provoke a few sideways double-take glances before I feel etiquette-bound to explain about them. I try to keep this short and sweet, desperately not wanting my health story to dominate the opening proceedings of any night out. Thirdly, and I've only tried this once, is to have a pair of 'normal shoes' that I exclusively wear indoors. This option requires me to contact the host beforehand to reassure them that – and as they don't seem to mind having their floors 'mopped' by friends' sweaty socks – my shoes are probably cleaner than their rugs and floorboards. The only time I tried this, a guest who knew me well enough and should've known better, approached me and explained that 'in our culture it is rude to wear shoes inside'. My inner monologue wanted to vocalise an extrapolated logic, 'in my culture it is rude to ask a person with no legs to leave their wheelchair by the door and spend the rest of their evening shuffling around on their arse'.

There were two particular parties which prompted me to become a permanent 'no shoes means no show' RSVPer for social occasions when strangers outnumber familiar faces. The first was a gathering at a former colleague's charming yet nooked and crannied apartment. I had no idea what to expect so really should've prepared better. Upon arrival, I could see a pile of shoes both inside and outside of the invitingly left-ajar threshold. Most people just kick off their shoes and saunter in, but that's a skillset my weakened ankle bones deny me. So the first attention-drawing thing I had to do was sit on my bum and unlace. Entering the flat I saw a large table and a number of chairs, although guests far outnumbered available seats. Everyone was standing and happily engaging anyway, so my co-attendee Sara suggested I snaffle a chair. So there I was, with my very own basecamp amidst a very mingle-y kinda throng. It was a highly sociable affair, and people were more than happy to introduce themselves, often launching into small talk with a name and a follow-up question as to how the host is known, before standard issue conversation commenced. It soon struck me that everyone had a far more interesting job and pivotal role in society than I, but they all did their best to diplomatically humour me in conversation despite the fact that I, as an English-language communications officer, could only really describe my occupation as 'writing in my native language better than my Swedish counterparts could write in their second language'.

It is hard to blend in as the only sitter in the room, acting like you're playing an imaginary game of musical chairs. After the third or fourth 'playful' 'Had a long day?' remark, or being discreetly asked if I was okay, I felt obliged to at least attempt a temporary period of standing. I surreptitiously used the back of the chair to partially support my weight and take a modicum of pressure off my feet. So while those I engaged with were chit-chatting, I was multitasking by both doing my best to be absorbed, amused and attentive, and at the same time working on my upper body strength as my puny biceps shuddered to support my puny body.

Mid-evening, I found myself talking to a woman called Lina. 'Brilliant', I thought to myself, earlier on in the evening I had met another Lina and if every woman here has the same name, other than Sara and the host, then that should relieve some social name-remembering anxiety. As I asked her a few tokenistic getting-to-know-you questions, she nodded and engaged in all the right places, but always with a slightly bemused and confused expression. It was as if she thought we'd met before, although I really could not place her for the life of me.

She told me she was an alumnus of the university I am employed by, and now worked as a boffin at a blood testing facility. As if that was not impressive enough, she then further revealed she was also in touch with her Sami roots (the indigenous population of the Sápmi region best known as 'Lapland' by those trying to contact Santa) by regularly heading north and helping to herd reindeer. There was a look of friendly concern as she relayed her tale. If I were anyone other than myself, I would have been utterly astonished by the fact that at one house party with about 50 guests there were two women with the same – to my ears rather unusual – name, both working as lab technicians and part-time reindeer herders/hunters. What were the odds, seriously? But I am not anyone else, I am me, and I now understood her bamboozlement. There was of course only one Lina, and only one blood-testing/reindeer herding woman in the room. It really could have been something as simple as her standing in a different light, her adding or removing a scarf, tying her hair up, or letting her hair down – it doesn't take much for my eyes to deceive me.

Soon followed the bespoke sinking feeling that I had made an incredible, massive twat of myself. I don't know what she must have thought of me. I wasn't slurring so I can't have seemed that drunk, although my arm muscles were sapped so I might have been swaying as I struggled to support my weight. With any luck, she probably just thought I had taken a bucketload of drugs, it was a party after all. And drugs are something I am often seen taking.

(At 09:30 and 21:30, seven days a week, a vibrating quack noise emanates from my phone. It is colloquially known as the 'pill alarm', and if I am not in the immediate vicinity of my phone at the time, the quacking is often chorused with a wife/friend/colleague beckoning me with the words, 'Your ducks are quacking'. If I am out and about, I produce a silver pillbox – a gift from my mother – and as discreetly as possible gulp down the pills – seven in the AM and eight in the PM – with a swig of water/tea/Riesling. I have become extremely adept at washing them down quickly, and if extreme needs-be, with no fluid whatsoever. In a social situation where it is impossible to do this unnoticed, I normally make 'a jocular thing' of taking them after having offered them around to anyone nearby.)

On that night, I was done. I couldn't take the shame any more than my body could take the strain. The combination of my impaired vision and fucked feet was proving too much. I headed for the pile of shoes and pathetically sifted through them trying to identify my own by touch rather than sight in the subdued lighting.

The second soul-crushing/social life defining event was a birthday-cum-flat-warming party. My connection to the hosts was tenuous to say the least. On top of that, most of my nearer and dearer peers have long since celebrated their 30th birthdays and probably most have moved into their home-for-life, which they will not leave until they relocate to a bungalow or a warden-assisted home for the elderly. I guess I felt 'pre-out of place' by demographics alone.

It was a swanky, open, spacious apartment and I could see, once again, as I sat on my arse to take my shoes off, that there was a kitchen table with chairs, some of which were occupied by others. Perfect. It might look a little rude to make a beeline for a chair, but a beeline was made all the same. Here would be my sanctuary for the night.

If only.

Soon after my friend Janni and I had made ourselves comfortable, a flurry of other guests arrived. Unlike Party No.1, we were, by good fortune, in a well-lit – for nibble prepping purposes – corner. This meant I could take a good mental picture of each guest as they hugged hello to the hosts.

An excitable conversation soon broke out around the table, as it was discovered one of the partygoers was a 'wallpaper designer'. This prompted the hostess to proudly announce that their newly decorated flat did indeed boast a wallpaper designed by the guest. All at once, the kitchen table was deserted as everyone temporarily decamped to an adjacent room. Everyone but me. Judging by the cooing of awe and appreciation, I can only imagine that the newly wallpapered interior was a hot contender for the next UNESCO heritage site or Turner Prize entry at the very least. How must I have looked? A blasé bastard, sat alone in that room, the only person who deemed the wallpaper unworthy of their admiration, or the only person who didn't want to risk a chronic foot fracture and possibly below the knee amputation? I doubt anyone jumped to the latter conclusion.

Janni had done a reconnaissance sweep of the flat and informed me that the room next to the kitchen boasted empty sofa space for three and was just a few hobbled steps away. Now armed with the knowledge I had gleaned from other shoeless house parties, I knew that staying too static and perched on a chair garnered unwanted questions and concern, so I made the move. The seating was more comfortable, but the lighting was far dimmer.

It was there that I became engrossed in conversation

with a Man&Woman comprised couple, the bloke half of the pairing was, other than Wallpaper Woman, one of the few guests who was not a classically trained musician (one of the hosts had worked as a music producer at my workplace, and her partner is an opera singer). I spent a good thirty minutes in his good-natured company, but after a while both Janni and I felt it was time to leave, what seemed to me, this clearly close-knit group of friends to their evening.

We re-shoed before a group of people who had gathered to bid us farewell. I could not see my hostess friend among them, but I spotted her opera singer partner, someone I had regrettably not had a chance to talk to the whole night. I started to profusely thank him for his hospitality, gushed about the new flat and its décor. I was more than audible to all, I was sincere. He was baffled ...

'That's not him', Janni discreetly heralded.

I would say that I wanted the world to open up, but my self-protectionism denies me that, I'd rather the whole building, the freshly-hipstered flat, and every soul in it bar me, with their newly forged who-the-fuck-is-this-guy memories, evaporated into a pile of dust and ash. The person I was thanking, congratulating, and praising was not the opera-singing co-host but rather the man I had just spent the last half an hour side-by-side chatting with. I was crushed beneath the weight of embarrassment and shame. Walking home, I vowed I'd never put myself in such a predicament again. And to this day, partly thanks to the corona pandemic, I do grant you, I haven't.

Do the biomedical scientist/reindeer herder, the opera singer, Wallpaper Woman, the genial, chatty bloke I shared a sofa with have a clue who I am? I doubt it very much, or rather I hope not because if so, then the only words which might spring to their minds upon that recollection are 'rude twat'. But I remember them, although not their faces obviously – if I could remember those, then these epically traumatising, embarrassing events would have never happened in the first place – but these defining moments are now part of my hardwiring, and I can't see them being eradicated any time soon. Evolution has taught us to 'fight' or 'take flight', but you don't need to do either if you 'don't turn up in the first place'.

*****

It is not that I am not a gregarious type of character, it is just that I cannot and will not put myself in that situation again. Not that get-togethers with familiar faces are any better – take a pre-pandemic Christmas office party, for example. The plan was innocuous enough: set up out-of-office auto-replies at our desks, drib and drab from our various corners over to a communal lounge area of the office, queue up at boss-bought boxes of booze, and enjoy a few parlour games before heading out for a Mexican dinner.

Before I knew it, we were being divvied up into teams and the instructions of a verbal-call and physical response game were explained. It was a game of speed and moderate agility which required short bursts of dashing. Nothing too excluding, just a short sprint which wouldn't daunt even the colleagues at the retirement end of the department's workforce.

What my feet can and cannot do can cause some confusion; it's all a question of skeletal deformity, misplaced tendons, and nerve damage. I can, for example, use them to walk with only a partial wonky gait, they can push pedals for miles and miles of cycling, they can even dance if I tone down the 'shapes' I once 'threw' pre-trauma, but I can't hop, skip, jump, and most certainly, I cannot run.

I managed to blend into the festive frolics by walking at pace rather than running, and taking advantage of my long, spindly legs and lunging steps to give the impression of genuine participation. But with every step I took, as the deformed ball of my foot crunched into the floor, all I could do was picture the tutting face of my foot specialist, Marita. I had spent a number of Christmases in plaster casts and hoped that this pre-dinner distraction was not to prompt the next. Fortunately, it didn't, but I did spend the rest of the evening in fear and checking my feet every time I went for a piss for any reddening and swelling – tell-tale signs I'd overdone it.

During summer months, give a socialising work group a wide-open space and some drinkies, and before you know it, some kind of ball kicking/catching/batting activity will ensue. My eyes are unable to focus on any fast-moving item flashing against the sky, thus prohibiting me from such pastimes. Being told I am in the 'red team' means nothing: 'red' to me is an indistinguishable blur of 'something' and 'blue' is an indistinguishable blur of 'something else', but if I don't see one by the side of the other, there is a good chance I cannot tell you which is which.

But my colleagues and society at large see me as they find me, and why wouldn't or shouldn't they? If I was my 2008-self and in a wheelchair, I have no question that my colleagues would accommodate that, but they know I cycle to work – just like everyone else – they see me work-

ing from a 'normal screen', just like everyone else. How
are they meant to understand the seemingly hypocritical
quirks of my disabilities? It is not as if I hand everyone
I come into contact with a 'Congratulations! You're now
working with an "Adrian"! Please read the following guidelines before use' set of instructions.

*****

And this is the world everyone was hankering after, was it?
The world the vaccination released back to the masses. A
world of buzzing workplaces, throngs of expectant queues
outside concert venues, rammed house parties, and roar-
ing and packed-to-the-rafters sporting arenas. I get the
appeal. I really do, but I've been burned and humbled by
that life – ableism runs far too readily through its veins –
and the pandemic gave me a glimpse into an alternative.
I've been a better English husband, Ogden the Cat owner;
I've been a more productive and conscientious employee,
and rather than being marginalised and compromised by
group dynamics, I've strengthened my friendships around
more bespoke 1-2-1 intimate interactions. Why would I so
keenly go back to that old life and leave a newfound con-
tentment behind?

Well, mainly because the doctor told me to, and if there
is one thing I like to think I've made abundantly evident,
it is that what the doctor tells me to do, I does. And maybe
I needed to make some kind of compromise with this em-
bryonating, vaccinated world, especially if I ever wanted
to see my friends and family in the UK ever again. I am
the polar opposite of any anti-vaxxer. It'd be hard to justify that stance with the pharmaceuticals I've injected into

myself over the years. I was, truth be told, a little hesitant about that needle popping the little bubble my life had become. But as my transplant consultant Kerstin had hoped, I was hurried to the upper echelons of the priority list, as was the cohabiting Swedish Wife.

On Thursday, March 18th, Tess and I headed off to Jab One. We filed in, were told to ditch our own face masks in favour of hospital endorsed ones, and before we had even completed the registration process, the well-oiled wheels of the Swedish administrative machine had already provided us with a date and time for Jab Two in exactly four weeks' time. We waited a minute or two, before being called to our respective booths where a prescribed measure of Moderna awaited us. I witnessed no palpable relief from anyone in the waiting room; no tears, no joy, no emotion, nada – it's the Swedish Way.

(If the Swedish Government tells its populace to 'jump', the populace not only asks, 'How high?' but it also clarifies when to jump, the preferred trajectory of the jump, and when to stop jumping. During the Italian lockdowns, videos of musicians performing on balconies went viral; in the UK – where a significantly smaller percentage of the population has attended a music conservatorium – people clapped, hollered, and banged wooden spoons on saucepans to show support for frontline workers. But in Sweden, adulation was far more muted; calls for higher wages for nurses drowned out the tokenistic clappers.)

On Thursday, April 15th, precisely four weeks later, Jab Two was administered. As a final nod to Sweden's now famed 'light touch' and rather ambivalent approach to the whole corona affair, I noted the nurse giving me my shot – in a room being used exclusively for highly-vulnerable transplant patients – was wearing his face mask over his mouth, but not over his nose.

*****

On that spring day, as Tess and I cycled home from hospital, with her left and my right arm starting to throb, just like they had after Jab One, we both had an underwhelming sense of, 'Well, I guess that's that then'. It was over a year since we had touched down back in Sweden after the trip to Thailand. Since then, we had lived the lockdown, caught the Covid, and now, received the remedy. But nothing really felt that different. Even after both the vaccines had kicked in and worked their medical magic, I knew I'd still be classified as vulnerable and that the vaccine would not protect me quite as well as it would protect others. I knew I'd still be, for a good while at least, working from home, still avoiding shops and social situations, and still not yet prepared to fly to my UK friends and family.

Is this it? My pandemic tale of woe concluding with more of an art house open-to-interpretation film ending rather than Tess and I embracing and walking towards a sunset Hollywood conclusion? What was left to do or say?

As it turned out, a lot – I've missed something rather pivotal out ...

Chapter 14
Flashback

So what was your worst Corona Horror Story© of the year 2020? That being the year, to date, most corona catastrophes have occurred.

Did you die? Or did your 35-year-old frontline paramedic son-in-law pass away? Maybe you've developed long Covid and haven't smelled your dinner or managed a flight of stairs without a breather since March 27th, 2020? Will you never walk again quite the same after your husband threw a hissy fit, grabbed a golf club that he'd not used since New Year's Day when he went for an early round, and pulverised your kneecap and crushed your lower femur just because you skipped ahead and watched an episode of Tiger King without him? Did you look on through a doubled-glazed window while you stood on the unkempt lawn of your dear, old, demented nan's nursing home as she faded away and died? Did you use a food bank for the first time? Lose your job, your business, your remnants of good mental health, your fight with addiction, or your will to live?

There really was a whole host of ways 2020 could have got ya, so many shades of personal hell, but as far as I was concerned, and now with the benefit of, albeit visually impaired, hindsight and perspective, I breezed through. 2021 though, that was the year that bit …

*****

I keep my pubic hair short short; less 'manscaped', more 'combine-harvested'. Anything remotely short and curly goes. I shave off any wispy strands of chest hair, hack away as the follicles thicken the lower the razor goes down my naval, and then practically crop my pubes to the core.

Some jump to the conclusion that anyone who invests so much time at the extreme edges of personal grooming does so in the pursuit of perversion, fetishism, or simply because they've been brainwashed by the hairless nubiles and libertines of the porn industry/contestants on dating reality telly shows.

For me, and quite possibly many like me, it is a personal hygiene-health thing. It is one element of keeping this body going for as long as I possibly can. And it all relates to the fact that I am constantly slathering on a layer of one type of gunk or another, pretty much day in and day out.

The cold, dry air of the winter months can dehydrate and crack the healthiest of skins, and with its multitude of scars, I consider my body 'pre-cracked'. I regularly snaffle Tess's body moisturisers, and if she is not within sniffing distance and I won't be rumbled by the fact that I reek of pink grapefruit, I'll plunder her stash of the body butter she reserves for a posh preen. My scars are prone to getting a bit itchy, and well-hydrated skin alleviates this. These scars do extend to the, what would normally be, hairier patches of the pubic region, so all hair there, goes.

During the dog days of the summer months, while my

skin can more readily hydrate from humidity, gunk comes in the form of suntan lotion. I am not a flaunter by nurture or nature, so my skin is rarely exposed, but when you are medicationally prone to skin cancer, you soon glean quite how futile clothes are when it comes to protecting you from the solar corona, even the crappy bit of the sun which shines on northern Europe. So while many will apply a slop of lotion to their face, neck, and ears, leaving t-shirts and other garb to do the heavy lifting/shading, I know that a cotton t-shirt offers only around a sun protection factor of seven – and my sun protection factor of choice is 50. When I apply, I apply. Not an inch of skin is left unprotected. I have enough potential health woes to worry about, I don't want to add skin cancer of the cock to the mix.

I am basically gunked in something sticky and icky more often than the average children's television presenter, or – if you are the type who still cannot disassociate buff, hairless bodies with sex – the average porn star after a day of filming.

With all the lotion, hydration, and protection my skin is treated to, my outer shell is normally as smooth as a freshly bathed and talced baby's bottom. Maybe it was because I was still insisting on outside coffees and catch-ups, still bicycling against Baltic bracing winds, but during the death throes of the winter months in early 2021, my skin finally gave in to the elements. My knuckles – which, even though gloved, take the brunt of the cold when I am out on my bike – went quickly from being smooth and silky to dry and flaky to weepy and bleed-y. More alarming, however, was a small patch of dry skin on my most prominent foot deformity.

While my bare feet do justify their medical description of 'acutely deformed', when shoed, I can mostly disguise this more freakish element of my physical appearance. Mostly, but not entirely. On the left side of my right foot is my original and most protruding bony bump. It extends out of my foot by about three centimetres and is about four centimetres in length. The bone is protected from the outside world and all its nastiness by a thin layer of skin. It was on the outermost apex of this bump where the dry skin had decided to set up base camp.

It seemed to me a minor ailment that I could DIY-handle with an extra splodge of my most potent moisturiser (used by Norwegian fishermen, the tube tells me), and an everyday band-aid for additional cushioning. Besides, at the time I noticed it, I was due to see Marita the Foot Lady the following week. It was a routine check-up on the hospital site which was, by happy coincidence, booked in an hour before Tess and I were due to have Jab One of our Covid vaccines..

I've seen the same Foot Lady for a few years now, and I like to think we have established quite a rapport. We know the basics of each other's family arrangements: I ask after her and her husband's new-found hobby of beekeeping, and she asks after Tess and her mushroom-foraging antics and whatever hare-brained plan I mentioned during my last appointment with her ('I'm gonna learn how to play the piano/write a book', et cetera, stuff like that).

She knows how much I care for my physical well-being, how mindful I am with both body and brain, and how I normally worry if even there is the remotest sign that there is something seriously awry ... perhaps, in her company, I am a 'foot fret-ishist'. Marita is seemingly well versed in controlling her facial muscles so as not to cause unnecessary alarm to a patient, a skillset I assume she has developed to lessen the panic when being presented with the occasional gangrenous and necrotic big toe. But she couldn't disguise this from me, a slight contort in her facial muscles and a look in her eyes. It was the look of a supressed 'oh, shit'.

The dry skin in question was, in effect, just a 'lid'. Beneath was an ulcer, the arch-rival to the lumped and bumped, nerve-damaged foot. Although shallow, it covered a big chunk of the thinly skinned deformity, and shallow was as deep as it was allowed to get. Any deeper, and there was a very real risk of it infecting bone. And infected bone is amputation territory.

Her panicked pupils were all the medical guidance I needed, to be honest. But to be on the safe side, she laid down the ground rules: walk as little as possible for as long as it takes. It came as a real blow, just as I was about to take my first step towards freedom, what with Jab One booked in just an hour after this appointment. Now I was being told not to take any steps at all.

I arrived at the vaccination site with a rather forlorn face, certainly not wearing an expression of joy and relief as one might possibly expect when your life is soon to be handed back to you with a measure of Moderna.

While this might be my path back to freedom, it was a path my foot specialist was now telling me I could no longer walk down. It was of some relief, however, that she was more than happy for me to cycle. And that's pretty much all I did. Just over a minute's walk from my front door was a newly opened café which a colleague and I had started to use on a regular basis for our coffee breaks instead of the now out-of-bounds office lounge. Despite it being a short walk from the kettle in my kitchen, the socially-distanced al fresco coffee was now a 15-second cycle away (although the faff of unlocking and relocking my bike took just as long as the short cycle itself). I did everything I could to keep the weight off that foot, while the healthcare system did its darndest to discover what had caused the initial injury. The dry skin being caused by the winter climes was a red herring, the injury was a result of something 'rubbing my bump'.

My foot appointments went from being once every two months to once a week. Every visit to Marita started with her whipping out a ruler to measure the size of the wound and ended with her handing me a bag of medical tape, plasters, and wound dressings. Meanwhile, the orthotics squad, who take charge of making my insoles, investigated and then created a new supportive sole. Sometimes the wound was smaller than it was at the previous check-up, and sometimes it was the same size. It was never getting bigger, which was the most important thing. Either way, Marita's instructions never wavered: I was not to walk until it was totally healed, and that could take months.

My appointments still seem to cluster up, not like the Dark Days of Dialysis when it felt like days not spent in a clinic or a day surgery were best described as 'weekends' – being ill really can be a full-time job. The morning after Jab Two, I had a routine blood test. Mild, flu-like side-effect symptoms had started to kick in around five hours after the needle retreated from its subcutaneous payload delivery point in my right arm. By the time I headed to bed, I was full-on shivery, although to my mind these were 'fake symptoms'. I figured I wasn't really ill, so when I woke up feeling even worse for wear than when I had nestled down, I braved the cycle to the hospital.

'No', I said, lying through my teeth when asked by the blood test centre's receptionist if I had any symptoms. The blood was taken, and not long after I was curled back up in bed in a foetal position, only moving for the rest of the day to put on an extra three hoodies, or to shed every layer due to the feverish heat burning inside me. A day later, I felt fine.

Two days later. My world caved in on itself.

*****

There is no question about it, even if I keel over in a coma tomorrow and spend the rest of my days on a what-kind-of-life-is-this support machine, I've been at the lucky end of the post-transplant survivor spectrum. The fact that no one can visibly see what I have been through (at least when I am fully dressed and wearing shoes), is nothing short of staggering. Medical science has brought me here, and the individuals who develop and deliver that science are keeping me here. I am watched like a hawk, but to be honest – all said and done – I am a fairly low maintenance patient. Sure, there's the occasional blip with the feet, but every blood and eye test and examination I've had post-transplant surgery, I've passed with flying (indistinguishable) colours.

Until that Monday. I had received Jab Two on a Thursday, I had taken my fever-wracked body for a blood test on the Friday, and on the following Monday my transplant consultant Kerstin had to do something she had hitherto never had to do.

Call me.

A general rule of thumb has always been, at least in my case, that a consultant only calls if there is an anomaly with a set of blood test results. Despite all that, I still felt no panic when I heard her calm and measured tone of voice. She was phoning to tell me that my results showed a raised level of infection biomarkers. Those 'fake symptoms' were maybe not as fake as I thought. I alerted her to the fact that I had been suffering the side-effects of Jab Two when the blood was drawn. This seemed to allay her; I then asked her if there was anything else.

There was.

The creatinine levels which indicate kidney function were alarmingly high. An early sign of the organ being rejected. The last time that level was that high was when the kidneys I was born with were both buggered.

I felt a cold rush of fear sweep through me. I asked if this could be a reaction to the vaccination and was met with a 'possibly'. But she was not done with the update yet. My pilfered pancreas was showing early indications it was now done with producing insulin to maintain my blood sugar levels and wanted to quit its role as one of my vital organs. 'We'll get some new blood tests done this week. I am sure everything will be fine', the consultant said.

Fine

F I N E

F   I   N   E

The word, the notion, the very concept of 'fine' dissipated as a tsunami of fear coursed through me. The floor fell away, the ground beneath the floor dissolved into nothingness. In an instant, I was left alone in a vacuum with only despair for company. I could feel the tip of the sword of

Damocles, which has hung low over my head ever since the transplant surgery, drop ever so slightly lower as its supporting horsehair rope started to fray. It was now brushing against my thinning curls, scratching the tip of my scalp.

There was nothing Tess or the handful of friends I told could do to distract me or reassure me. I could maybe understand why the vaccination had prompted a spike in whatever it is blood boffins use to measure infection levels, but how could the jab have any effect on my kidney and pancreas function? It just made no sense to me, and so my Cynical Sense once more worked its 'magic' and concluded that the timing of the jab and the sudden onset of organ failure was down to nothing more than coincidence.

The routine blood test which had led to this catastrophic culmination of the life I had rebuilt, was carried out (as was always the case) a week before my three-monthly check-up. This appointment is normally made up of a friendly chat, Kerstin the Consultant telling me that all my blood test results were 'excellent', a blood pressure test, a bit of poking and prodding, and, on one occasion, a finger up a bum (her finger up my bum, I hasten to add).

This time, however, with my pallid complexion and my face frozen in fear, it was obvious from the offset that this was not going to be one of those casual and convivial consultations. It was a Wednesday morning, and I had now been festering in a fear-laced depression for 48 hours. I had tried to distract myself with long bike rides, but I could not outride my thoughts.

If this really was the end of my post-transplant Life 2.0, then what else did it mean? Back on dialysis? I am sure I had read somewhere that once you've had a stint on peritoneal dialysis – the one you can hook yourself up to in your own home – you cannot go back to it; the only option is therefore haemodialysis – an enforced option that would require every other day me going to a special unit for hours on end. And how long would I be on that for? Quite likely, the rest of my life (which if multiple organ failure was to play out, would probably not be that long).

And how long would it take for the rest of my body to follow suit? My eyesight is dependent on well-balanced blood, and my nervous system – already pushed to its limits – would take a pounding. Oedema, nausea, comas, blindness, wheelchairs ... they all felt like 'the next step' in my medical journey.

And what of my UK family and friends? They were all so pivotal during my first bout with ill health. I had not seen them now for well over a year, and it was starting to dawn on me that I may never see them again. A combination of my potential medical needs and a pandemic would make certain of that. Was my brain jumping to the most cataclysmic conclusions? Possibly, but unless you've been through what I've been through, may I suggest you don't judge me on that. It is not as if I don't have a wife, a life, and friends who are becoming dearer and dearer to me as each day passes here in Sweden, but the thought of not seeing my mother, my brother, and my UK friends ever again, was crushing my very being.

While Tess had been doing her best to reason with logic in a bid to calm my nerves, I had no problems pulverising any positivity or optimism with acerbic, cynical vigour. Work rumbled on, my unwitting colleagues had no inkling of what was going on down this end of the Zoom meeting: 'Do you think that is a good idea, Adrian?', a middle manager rhetorically queried. Like I could give a flying fuck about a communication plan which, to my mind, now had a life expectancy longer than my own.

On top of all this, I was still under stern instruction from Marita the Foot Lady to exercise extreme caution with everything I did. A problematic foot, some dodgy blood test results, it was all starting to feel very déjà vu-y. It was obvious to Kerstin that this was playing heavily on my mind, and once she was done with her routine poke, she sent me off with some mild-mannered reassurance ('I'm sure it will probably be *fine*' – that word again) and the paperwork I needed for a new set of blood tests – they were to be done first thing the following day. After another sleepless night, I cycled back to the hospital for the deciding blood to be drawn.

I hadn't been eating well for a few days now; I felt the encroaching presence of the anorexia nervosa I suffered as a student every time I took a mouthful. Despite that, the fact that I cannot eat before a morning blood test meant some form of sustenance was required upon return from the blood testing hospital department. While the bread toasted, I checked my phone, which I had just noticed had been set to silence. There was a missed call from a withheld number.

I scrolled back in my phone to see that the last time I had been called from a withheld number was when Kerstin had called on the Monday. I did not think it was possible for my despair to envelop me further, but now it was crushing me. If it was her, then why was she calling me so soon after the blood tests? How bad must they have been for her to take such prompt action? This was it. I was fucked.

As the toaster ejected the produce of its morning labours, the phone rang again. It was Kerstin, and before

I got a word in, I heard, 'You're okay', followed swiftly by 'Your bloods are back to normal'. I can only assume she had chased up these results in a bid to put me out of my misery as soon as was humanly possible. I thanked her, ended the call, and crumpled into a sobbing mess; Tess raced to embrace me as I told her the news. The rest of the day was spent lying on the sofa, where I broke out into intermittent bouts of weeping as my body convulsed as if trying to rid itself of the trauma that had been building up inside it for four days now. The toast never got eaten, but my appetite was back with vengeance by dinnertime.

I can hardly talk – or indeed write, as I have just now discovered – about that week without welling up. I would investigate post-traumatic stress disorder to see if I have any of the symptoms, but I really don't want to add any other ailment to my ever-fattening medical records. I've never slept quite the same since though, I can tell you that, such was the trauma and subsequent ripple effect of those four days.

*****

So, that's my very own, uniquely bespoke Covid Horror Story.© And I hope it is the last. It certainly made actually contracting Covid pale into insignificance by comparison. As I type, the virus variants are slowly infecting their way through the Greek alphabet, the next letter seemingly more spreadable but less potent than the last. Rolling news seems to be distracted by something even more dystopic and perhaps, right now, you are reading this by torchlight in a bunker. My scientific-free best guess is that, unless the Omega variant has grown a new tentacle-like spike with fangs, a spike that can burrow into our marrow and make the infected a blood-thirsty zombie who will yoink out the brains of anyone who gets between them and a freshly filled supermarket shelf of toilet paper, we're probably through the worst of this.

Already I can hear people discuss the pandemic in the past tense, rejoicing in whatever it is they deem 'normality'. I can't help but think of pub table discussions in five years' time, when people will look back upon this period of history. Some will be wearing their rose-tinted glasses, harking on about the joys of a lazy lockdown or the 'blitz spirit' which saw 'us Brits' through this harrowing mini-era. ('Blitz' talk was thin on the ground in my family, seeing as my London-living great grandparents were both squished to death in the single most deadly strike of that particular bombing campaign, but I've seen photos of them, and they did not look like the types who'd equate 'blitz spirit' with sitting on their bums all day shovelling Pringles down their gullets). I cannot underestimate how difficult life was for so many people forced into lockdown, but I do take quiet offence by comparing that with the resolve it must've taken to live through six months of sustained bombing. Sure, it might've been tough waking up to discover your neighbour had been rushed to hospital gasping for breath, but not as tough as waking to find your neighbour's head on your front lawn after he was blown to smithereens.

Maybe others around that pub table will quietly reflect on the loss of a grandparent. Perhaps others might still be convincing themselves that the whole thing was a global conspiracy engineered by Bill Gates in cahoots with 'the Jews'. I imagine, if the conspiracies play out, come the

Great Reset, I'll be among the first to be cast to the gutters now my foreskin has been lopped off, rendering me genitally Jewish. But by then, I suspect, there will be a new 'chamber' and the 'echo' will be resonating with a new line in bonkerism.

But what of the Shielders and the Vulnerables? What of our plights? What will our 'new normal' herald? Some of us have made it this far, are we now to be thrown back to, in my personal experience, an ableist society?

I am not expecting an ableist-free world to rise from the ashes of a Covid-ravaged world, and I am not going to suggest that society bend over backwards to meet the whims of my disease-wracked body, but if we can learn one thing, then can it be to appreciate quite how 'vulnerable' so many of us are?

That cuddly uncle of yours, the one who wore that 'Beer Built This' t-shirt? Not quite so cuddly now is he? Now he's decomposing skin and bones and six feet under. Did you know Sharon in accounts was an asthmatic? She probably didn't feel any need to mention it until the paramedics turned up at her house after a panicked call from her fella. Sad how they turned up too late, mind. The guy who used to ref the junior football on a Saturday morning, dead. Dicky ticker, apparently, although you'd never have guessed by the way he charged up and down that pitch. It's a shame it has taken so many tragedies for us to wake up. Please – all this 'lanky prick who moved to Sweden' wants is for us not to fall back to sleep.

Pre-Covid, every time I'd hear someone sneeze in my near vicinity, I'd await the first coming-down-with-something symptoms, having no way of knowing whether the airborne infection-riddled particles of snot had penetrated my immune system and I'd get a mild cold which would take me out of commission for a week, or whether that globule of goo you just jettisoned into the atmosphere could be the first step in a chain reaction which renders me dead.

There have always been a select few who acknowledge my vulnerableness and stay well clear of me when they fear their flu could be my fate, but we live in a world where young children are awarded and praised for full attendance at school. Does it make you a proud parent knowing that you are installing in that child the same mentality that will make them 'soldier on' and head to the office despite the fact that they look like partially defrosted Death. And the risible notion of 'man-flu', if someone is ill, can we stop with the sick shaming?

If all the scientists and Hollywood B-movie makers are correct, then this probably won't be our last showdown with a killer bug. And you never know, as you read this, there might be a bird – one of those you've seen on a David Attenborough wildlife documentary, one of those birds with a flamboyant mating dance – taking a poo on an unknowing cameraperson's ham and cheese sandwich. Perhaps that poo in that lunch will trigger a whole new virus. And will that virus hone in on 18- to 25-year-old Insta-influencers or Premier League football players? No, it'll go for the same ol' targets all viruses go far – those with underlying health issues.

Sooner or later, something will kill me. So do me a favour, make sure that something is not a someone, and that someone is not *You*.

Epilogue

I did eventually get back to the UK. I flew in on August 6th, 2021, for a two-week and one day mad-dash catch-up. I had allowed for a quarantining period of a week, that being the rule when I booked the ticket, but it wasn't the rule by the time I landed; so were the ever-shifting sands of the UK's corona restrictions.

I had not, until the point of entering the airport of departure, ever worn a face mask for longer than a hospital appointment. So, upon arrival and with my specs steamed up, I got my first taste and (an even more) blurred view of life emerging from the latest lockdown in a country still fresh from 'Freedom Day'. Mum met me at the local village's railway station, where I've been dropped off and picked up for as long as I can remember. 'Do we hug?' I cautiously asked. We hugged. And we are not a family of huggers. Mum looked exactly the same as she did the last time I saw her – which, thanks to video chat tech, was only a week earlier.

I am not sure what I was expecting to see as I gazed out of the car window on the way home, both of us having shed our masks. There were no packs of stray, pandemic-purchased and newly abandoned dogs running loose, or solitary cyclists on endless miles of open road pointlessly wearing face masks. Instead, I was met with undulating crop fields of varying colours sweeping off into the horizon, and the miles of country lanes that thread through those fields bore no scars of the world's recent history. Everything felt normal enough to me.

The day after I had arrived, I was lying on the sofa reading. Mum was sat nearby also engrossed in a book, and Barry was fixated on the screen of a handheld games console like a monosyllabic teenager. We'd all been there in our respective little world for some time. The occasional chirp of a nesting bird in the garden was all that ever punctuated the silence. It was all rather pleasantly subdued and serene. Mum looked up from her thriller and said, 'Imagine doing only this for three months'. The idea that endless days were spent doing this and only this flipped my mind-mood from calm to Kafkaesque in an instant. Everything felt a little less normal to me.

The newfound common courtesy seemed to be to send a photo of a recently taken negative-revealing antigen Covid test the morning of the day you were due to meet anyone. And the first person I sent that photo to was, of course, my friend since the age of three, Karen. She replied with a matching photo green-lighting our impending catch-up in the café of a local farm shop.

I can meet Karen presented in a number of dynamics: herself and her husband; herself, her husband and their two children; herself, her husband and a handful of mutual friends; and any combination of the aforementioned pairings and groupings. But it was only after I met her on that Sunday afternoon that I truly understood the dynamic I had missed the most. Just the two of us.

Our friendship was forged as teenagers, normally perched on her cabin bed, under a giant poster of Bruce Willis next to recently attended gig flyers that were starting to completely plaster over the love heart-patterned wallpaper that Bruce left exposed. That's where our bond truly started, and that is where I was transported back to as we giggled and gossiped through our reunion.

A few days later I was in Cambridge and out for dinner and drinks with another nearest and dearest, Emily – someone I've known since I was sixteen. A sturdy gent stood astride the bar's entrance, and before we crossed the threshold, he explained the establishment's current corona guidelines, to which we listened attentively: 'Right. You'll need to go in, head to the bar, order your drinks, pay for your drinks and then find somewhere to sit.' From where I was standing, it felt like the UK had suffered collective amnesia. He stopped short of telling us we'd have to 'transfer the fluids from the glass to our mouths' and later 'direct our piss into the porcelain bowls in the side rooms' once the fluids had worked through our systems. As far as I was concerned, this is how I'd been ordering drinks ever since I had fake ID.

I was finally getting a whiff of what life might have been like for me had I experienced a UK-flavoured pandemic. A few days later I was back in the same city and waiting to get picked up by a group of old friends. They pulled over in a nearby bus stop, and I hopped in. Just like Karen, I hadn't seen Neil, Danny, Nick and Amy for eighteen months. 'So, how was your pandemic?' I queried within seconds. 'Fine,' were the respective replies, and not one corona-related word was uttered for the next eight hours of blissful and joyous reunion as we ate, drank, and played the fool in pub gardens and parks.

Toby, Aine, Daniel, Andrew, Clare, Tim, Helen, a brother, a sister-in-law, a cousin and his family, godkids and their siblings – the reunions came thick and fast. These people are the reason I'll always have one mutilated foot in the UK and the other in Sweden. I've gotten used to the fact that I have a wife and a life in one country but an overwhelming sense of belonging in another. I rather enjoy the fact, indeed. And this trip felt especially special.

*****

During the process of writing this book, there was a sense of wariness every time I used an expletive, referred to masturbation, pooing in a bin bag, or indeed when I wrote a 5000-word long chapter primarily focusing on my penis. I knew there would be every chance that some of my friends' parents would read this, and some of those parents are in turn friends with my mother. 'I read Adrian's book', they might politely enthuse to my mum, but with the subtext of 'he writes an awful lot about his willy, doesn't he?'. My mum would know what they've read, and the rest of the conversation would be a blur to her as her inner self crumples with embarrassment.

I had thought by this stage of the writing process, I'd be done with all the foul language and sexual references, but it might be that I've ended up having to save the best/ worst and most aggressive tone for last. I never intended this book to be so profanity-laden, and I certainly sidestepped the extreme end of the expletive spectrum. Until now. Or rather until I returned to the office in September 2021 to meet a woman called Anna and left the office with the words 'what an absolute, total and utter thoughtless fucking cunt' reverberating around my brain.

Anna was interviewing for a job as the maternity cover for one of my closest colleagues, and I was part of the interview process. She was the most qualified, and accordingly got the position. It was only a matter of time before I felt compelled to deliver my well-rehearsed spiel about my eyesight which has caused, and continues to cause, so much embarrassment: 'I will never knowingly ignore you, but ...' is the opening line.

(It is practically an every-other-day occurrence that a colleague or a friend will tell me they waved at me as I cycled past them. 'You must have been in your own little world. You were looking right at me' is their follow-up, which triggers my here we go again self-loathing.)

My 'spiel' is often met with, I presume, an intended considered and comforting counter-utterance of, 'Oh, I am the same. Blind as a bat without my glasses'. Anna, however, saw this as an opportunity to mention her own chronic health issues.

And what issues they are. Her own guts and gory bits, while not as messed up as mine, are certainly more messy than most. This conversation started a connection which bolstered us into a bond, and within months she was not only a colleague but also a chum and a confidante, depending on whether we are in the office, in our favourite restaurant, or in deep conversation.

Chum, colleague, confidant, but most certainly not a 'cunt'. No, it was the 'returning to the office' which jettisoned that word from the gutter of my brain to the mutterings under my breath. Truth is, I was not returning to the office I had left, as our department had relocated mid-pandemic. To my absolute horror, the office was now, for me, a veritable assault course-cum-death trap: the fabric of the office chairs was, to my undiscerning eyes, the exact colour as the carpet.

Whether the f-ing and the c-ing were directed at whomever the office planner was who made such an ableist oversight, or to myself when for the first time I cluttered into a roguely placed chair I am unsure.

The colour coordination is to such an extreme that I could actually put a hand on the back of the chair and still have to make my best educated guess, based on the curve of the head rest, as to where I should navigate my arse. Over the weeks and months I perfected the art of sitting down, it is not foolproof, but at least any colleague in earshot is now more than aware of this issue as I make my feelings of frustration audibly and aggressively clear.

It is hard to know how such an issue can be remedied: replace a couple of hundred square metres of carpet or replace 40-odd chairs? Personally I don't want the fuss, but I am no shrinking violet, and I know the higher-ups are working to resolve the issue. How many offices around the world are there where others face a similar plight but who may not have the same voracity of voice or the same compassion of their colleagues? There's a lot of ableist f-ing c's out there, I know that for sure.

*****

As the writing of this book progressed, it occurred to me that a tying-up of loose ends final chapter might be comprised of a number of communications I could set up between myself and some of the unwitting characters who feature in these pages. Beyond family, friends and the legions of healthcare professionals I have name-checked, there are a number of unknowns who've had either an incidental or direct impact on my life. Of course, the contents of the final chapter 'Flashback' took precedence, and I hope you understand why. Either way, the more I pondered on my original idea, the more I self-thwarted it.

Take, if you will, 'Pharmacy Girl'. What good would come of trying to contact a woman I had met just a handful of times to confess that the man who she would know as the patient with dark brown, matted and greasy hair, was nil-by-mouth, once shat his bed, and had to piss into a bag actually had a 'bit of a crush' on her? I imagine the most likely outcome would be a restraining order. Besides, how on earth could I track her down? I typed 'pretty pharmacist working in Addenbrooke's Hospital in 2009' into Google. I know I was on a lot of pain relief back then, but I am fairly sure my crush was not on a 52-year-old Australian bloke called Terry Pretty, as the search engine revealed.

And what of Nemesisson, the man working for the same organisation as I who had unwittingly led to a dent in my mental health after I followed his every physical activity over a five-week period? As a member of a two thousand-strong workforce, all of whom have a profile on our website, he'd not be hard to trace. But how on earth do you broach that subject? How would it make you feel if some random bloke from another department presented you with such a stalker-y tale? And were the odds I might share an elevator with the guy in the future high enough for me to risk it? No.

The only people I felt comfortable enough to approach were two of the party guests who, unbeknown to them, were partly yet blamelessly responsible for me never attending a Swedish house party again. What with the respective hosts of the two parties in question being mutual friends with the guests and myself, they were relatively easy to trace.

Lina is the biomedical scientist/reindeer herder who I had mistakenly spoken to twice without me knowing it was the same person. When presented with my account of that evening's events, she had a patchy memory of the incident but gave an understanding reply: 'I don't think you're a twat. Life is complicated and I'm not the shiny centre of it.' She also forwarded to me a photo of herself, wearing a high vis gilet, standing next to a reindeer. If only she had brought both that cloven-hooved beast and worn that reflective attire to the party, I'm sure I'd have had no issues identifying her, but my guess is that if one isn't even allowed to wear shoes in a Swede's home, one sure as hell can't get away with hooves.

'Wallpaper Woman' – known more widely, as it turns out, as Sara – was the guest at the last house party I have ever attended. Still. She was the lady whose daily toils I had snubbed after failing to traipse my Quasimodo'ed feet to an adjacent room to admire the wallpaper she herself had creatively conjured. 'I do remember you!' she wrote, diplomatically, I'd wager, failing to state what she remembered me for. 'However, I don't remember that you didn't look at the wallpaper at the party. I'm a bit embarrassed, I sound very into myself', she continued.

But then she revealed this: 'I actually have a chronic condition myself that's not visible from the outside that I have to deal with in many social situations'. It was a revelation that evoked in me – possibly incredibly selfishly – a twisted, imagined world in a parallel universe where everyone had a disability of one description or another, whether visible, hidden, or disguised. What a truly understanding and empathetic world that would be! That's a bizarre sentiment to end an epilogue on, but here it ends.

Acknowledgements

This was meant to be for the 'crew' that helped this book come to be, as I think enough praise is lavished on the 'cast' of the book in the book itself. But then, as I pondered on all the people who have supported this writing project, I realised that many of the crew made cameos as cast members.

Mum, Tess … you've read the book. You know what you've done and continue to do for me.

I've only used first names in the book, apart from some of the doctors (I changed the name of the doctor I didn't like for obvious legal reasons). It did occur to me that there are three Daniels, but you can probably work out which Daniel you are by context and location, although if none of you want to lay claim to being the fart-obsessed, alpha-male Daniel, I get it.

Anyway, here is a chronological account of how I abused my friendships over the last year or two in the form of a list of those without whom I can honestly say this book would not have come to fruition. Let's start with Ellen Albertsdóttir, a former colleague and now current friend, whose passing comment – as mentioned in the foreword – got this book-shaped ball rolling.

Next up, Toby Allanson and Emma Sleightholm, who both acted as counsel and critic as I dragged them kicking and correcting me through the writing process. After the Swedish Wife had read a completed chapter, it was Toby and Emma who proffered up feedback.

'Savage' by surname and 'savage by editing nature', Carolyn gave each chapter an eagle-eyed edit – I will forever be grateful for her word nerdering. Also, Will 'the neigh-bour' Gray illustrated both the front and back cover, for which he only accepted the payment of a cream bun and two bottles of plonk. That process did, however, involve me stripping to the waist in his study so he could take photos of my scarred-to-smithereens torso. Whether Will has profited from those photos by uploading them to a niche fetish website I have no idea, but good luck to him if he has.

For the purposes of determining whether the 'foreigners will get this book', Johanna Svensson and Anna Jaakonaho were among the first to read an early draft from cover to cover. Both came back with scribbles on post-it notes and photos of pages on phones highlighting 'you're-gonna-wanna-change-that' faux pas.

Johanna and Anna I know through my job at Malmö University and, in a roundabouts kind of way, I should thank my managers there too. Some might consider me a 'kiss-ass' for praising my managers, but as Ingrid Persson and Charlotte Löndahl Bechmann both know, I'd edit that to be 'kiss-arse', given part of my role is to correct any American spellings to British spellings. I started working there in 2015 as 'the English chap in the communications office', and the job has both empowered and enriched my post-transplant life. Ingrid's face practically lit up with glee when I warned her there was a chapter where I imply she might have inadvertently tried to kill me by encouraging her department to exercise. And ever since, she has shown what appears to be a very genuine interest in the progress of the book. Charlotte, a published travel guidebook writer no less, would always add an extra 'And how is it going with the book?' section to our 1-2-1s. Never forced nor faked. I thank you both for nurturing an inclusive and creative work environment, at least as far as my 'errant English bloke in the office role' is concerned. Also, apparently neither of you noticed how many reams of printer paper we got through at the same time I was completing my first two drafts. And thanks also to manager Maria Crona for sorting out that fucking matching chair and carpet nightmare.

I never made any secret of this side project from chums and colleagues, and I received nothing but enthusiasm and excitement. It never failed to motivate. If there was any unfaltering ray of sunshine, which could flummox even NASA's top solar–stellar scientist, then it must surely be Selina-Marie Voss. So keen was she to buy a copy for herself, and by the sounds of it, for a host of friends, that I was forced to throw her the occasional chapter to quell her. All that did was fuel enthusiasm.

The final, final, final draft (after I had tampered with Carolyn's fine work) was completed by Janet Feenstra. If you found any typos or grammar or spelling mistakes, then blame my final jiggery-pokery edits and not Carolyn or Janet. The accompanying website was built by Janni Karlsson, who used both her web-brain and her cringe-brain as I made suggestions as to how it might look.

And lastly, it is only thanks to the medical staff of King's College Hospital in London, Addenbrooke's Hospital in Cambridge, and Skånes universitetssjukhus in Malmö, Sweden, that I am here today. I have passed through so many caring hands – from professors to porters – since my health started to dwindle, but there is no question that these have been the key players:

Professor Michael Edmonds
Mr Martin Snead
Professor Gavin Pettigrew
Doctor Kerstin Westman

It is hard to express the emotions one feels for such medical professionals: I've been part of their daily to-do lists, but they will forever be part of my life – a life they've either saved or are keeping functioning.

Although those professionals may have medically saved my life, it was of course both my father (who passed away in 2003) and my mother who gave me life in the first place. And not just life, but a can-do, should-do, must-do, will-do ethic, without which I would not have been able to go through what you now know I have been through. And it is with that ethic that I have then gone on to rebuild my life, meet my wife, hold down a job, cycle the length of Sweden on an 85-year-old bike for no real reason whatsoever, and write a book. This book.

Thanks all.

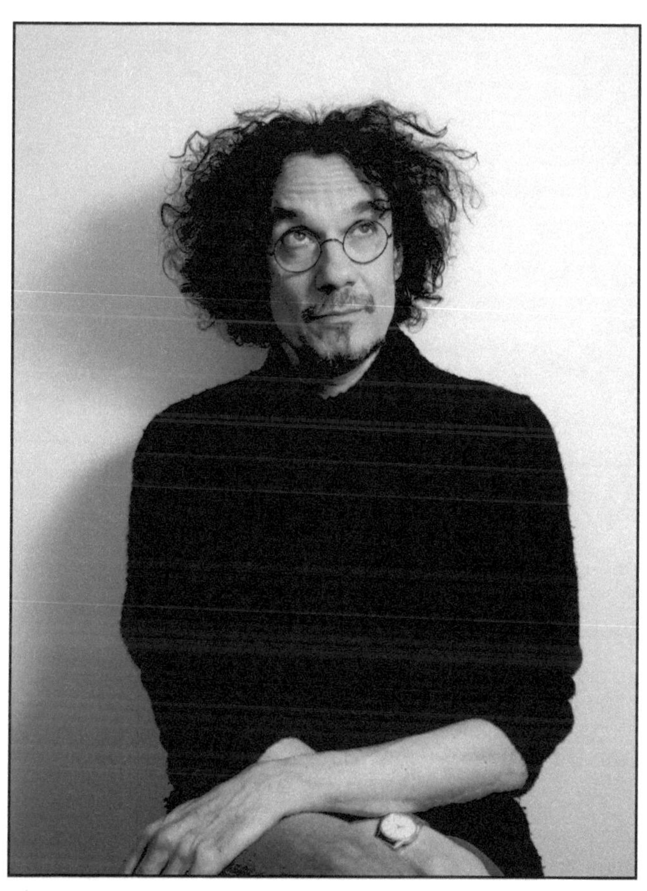

Also by the same author:

Zilch, nada, nix. This is the only book he's written
... so far.